ROAD TO
ANANDA

Simple Guide to the Endocannabinoid System,
Hemp Phytocannabinoids/CBD and Your Health

ROAD TO ANANDA

Simple Guide to the Endocannabinoid System,
Hemp Phytocannabinoids/CBD and Your Health

Carl Germano, CNS, CDN
INTRODUCTION BY
Dr. Raphael Mechoulam
"Father of Cannabinoid Medicine'
FOREWARD BY
Dr. Joseph Mercola

Illustrated and Designed by
David Marshall

An award winning graphic designer, illustrator, and children's book author.
David works to introduce health and wellness education in the science of
biology, nutrition, and emotional wellness.

Book Design by David Marshall
Cover Illustration by David Marshall

Library Congress Cataloging-in-Publication Data
Germano, Carl
ROAD TO ANANDA
Simple Guide to the Endocannabinoid System
Hemp Phytocannabinoids/CBD and Your Health

ISBN 978-0-578-44792-6

Printed in the United States of America

First Edition

TABLE OF CONTENTS

Dedication

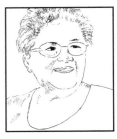
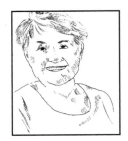

Franes Surdi   *Anne Carbone*

To my mother Frances and Aunt Anne – thank you for your endless love, for always being there, and unwavering guidance you both have provided to me.

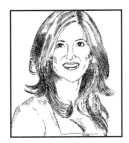

Debby Stromberg

To Debby – thanks to my life partner whose unconditional love, encouragement, emotional sustenance and unquestioning support has been my nourishment in life and beacon for renewed love.

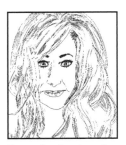

Beata Jerdrzejewska

To Beata – thank you for being my friend and colleague and providing me the opportunity of a lifetime. Your generosity, support, and trust is unwavering and I am eternally grateful to you.

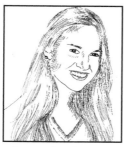
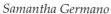
Samantha Germano

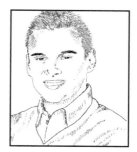
Grant Germano

To my son Grant and daughter Samantha – You are not just my children that I am immensely proud of, but rather my reason for living and my source of joy and happiness.

Foreward

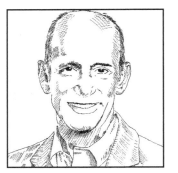

In ancient times, the depression-pain combination was treated through the use of extracts of the Cannabis sativa plant, commonly known as marijuana. Historically, marijuana use dates back to 2000 BCE. Surprisingly, both humans and animals alike naturally synthesize endogenous cannabinoids, chemical compounds.

The prohibition of cannabis in the middle of the 20th century halted cannabis research. For far too long the prospect of understanding the importance of hemp (Cannabis sativa) and its active components, phytocannabinoids, has been shadowed by calculated misinformation that's been force fed, and the ensuing stigma attached to the plant.

There is a clear distinction between marijuana and hemp – both legally and phytochemically. While both hemp and marijuana are from the same species of Cannabis sativa, Federal and state laws define hemp as cannabis sativa plants that have less than 0.3 percent THC. It's taken 70 years, but hemp finally had its "day in court" in December, 2018 when President Trump signed the Hemp Farming Act into law, which removed it from the Controlled Substances Act. Thankfully, the stigma and dark days of hemp are now over. The opportunity to open the doors for further research into the clinical potential of hemp-derived phytocannabinoids and their effects on the most important physiological system in the body, the Endocannabinoid System (ECS), is upon us.

In the "Road To Ananda," you will find valuable insights and current scientific and medical information available about the ECS. While many textbooks and studies exist on this subject, this book will provide a simplified vision of the inner workings of a remarkable medical discovery; the role the ECS has in your health and disease.

The 1990's were an important decade of discovery for the ECS and at the helm of this unearthing was the work of Dr. Raphael Mechoulam, Hebrew University, Jerusalem. As a functional medicine practitioner, his work inspired me to further my own understanding of the ECS, and its potential implications for clinical treatment.

Thanks to Dr. Mechoulam's work and many other published research studies conducted at prestigious institutions around the world, we are getting closer to unraveling the enormous potential of how supporting the ECS can impact your health.

The dawning support and appreciation among health care practitioners of the role of the ECS as a master regulator of all physiological functioning, and usefulness of hemp phytocannabinoids to support it represents a major paradigm shift in botanical medicine. We are now able to harvest information from the front lines of science and medicine on how best to achieve optimal health through supporting the ECS.

Nutritional and botanical science is barely more than a century old. Yet today, a major breakthrough in natural medicine has occurred through our understanding of how hemp derived phytocannabinoids assist in nourishing and supporting the ECS. Equally, we are now grasping the incredible role of how the ECS keeps you in balance (homeostasis/adaptogenic) and its association with disease when it is not properly maintained.

This includes conditions such as migraines, fibromyalgia, irritable bowel syndrome and many others. Essentially, your ability to maintain optimal health rests on your responsibility to become informed about the ECS and its involvement in the underlying causes of many degenerative diseases. This book by Carl Germano is a brilliant start!

From the earliest moments of development, to the last stages of life, your ECS is involved in constant mass communication with every organ system in your body, acting as the conductor in a symphony. Biologic communication between all of your organs and the ECS relies on messenger molecules the ECS produces (endocannabinoids), and the doorways (receptors) on each and every cell that accept them.

Once endocannabinoids enter your receptors, they seek to maintain homeostasis through influencing important regulatory mechanisms that govern major physiological processes which include but are not limited to:

- Chronic stress and anxiety conditions
- Obesity and insulin sensitivity
- Nervous system health
- Pain and Inflammatory cycles
- Heart and blood vessel health
- Cancer
- Insomnia
- Eye Health
- Bone repair/formation
- Reproductive system health

Homeostasis is critical to your body and your ability to adapt to the daily bombardment of the environment and stress. So, when your ECS is functioning properly you enter a state of balance, health, and well-being. When the ECS is not functioning properly, illness ensues.

The endocannabinoids we produce in the body are crucial to bioregulation. Their main role is in cell-signaling, and, because of their fat soluble nature, their main actions are limited to paracrine (cell-to-cell) or autocrine (same cell) signaling, rather than systemic effects.

With the current opioid crisis the US is in, it is helpful to realize that supporting the ECS, cannabis, and hemp phytocannabinoids have been shown to be very useful in the management of chronic pain. The mechanisms of the analgesic and anti-inflammatory effects of phytocannabinoids include inhibition of the release of neurotransmitters and neuropeptides from presynaptic nerve endings, modulation of postsynaptic neuron excitability, activation of descending inhibitory pain pathways, and reduction of neural inflammation. Modulation of your ECS system may be a cure for more chronic neurologic and immune conditions. Research in animal models suggests the possible use of cannabinoids as anticancer drugs.

When you don't have enough endocannabinoids around to participate in adaptation and equilibrium the ECS is responsible for, an endocannabinoid deficiency state can ensue. The consequences of an ECS deficiency most likely plays a major contributing role in the etiology of many degenerative diseases, especially those that are neurological and inflammatory in nature.

Thankfully, hemp serves as a repository for active phytocannabinoids that can be suitably used to support the ECS or used in an overall protocol for treatment. While high doses of cannabinoids have been benficial in clinical trials, even small doses of hemp phytocannabinoids help support proper functioning of the ECS and can serve as a daily balancer for your body.

Hopefully you will use the Road To Ananda as a valuable resource in your first step toward exploring the remarkable inner workings of the ECS, and the enormous potential that hemp derived phytocannabinoids have to optimize and improve your health.

Dr. Joseph Mercola
Functional Medicine Physician

Acknowledgments

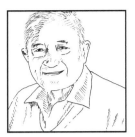

To Dr. Mechoulam – thank you for your esteemed work and illustrious career which has provided me the inspiration to write this book. I am deeply grateful for your contribution to the book and your tremendous influence you have made in science & medicine. My intent is for this book to serve as a conduit to help people outside of the scientific community understand and appreciate the remarkable achievements you have bestowed on us. Dr. Raphael Mechoulam is the esteemed professor of Medicinal Chemistry at the Hebrew University of Jerusalem, Israel. Best known for his work on the isolation and synthesis of THC (tetrahydrocannabinol) and the endocannabinoids anandamide and 2-AG, he has been called the "Father of Cannabinoid Research" by many. Dr. Mechoulam has published over 350 scientific articles and is the recipient of numerous awards and honors including the European College of Neuropsychopharmacology Lifetime Achievement Award, the International Cannabinoid Research Society Lifetime Achievement Award, the Eicosanoid Research Foundation Lifetime Achievement Award, and the American Botanical Council Norman Farnsworth Excellence in Botanical Research Award.

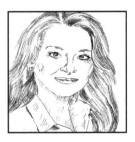

Dr. Magdalena Bujalska-Zadrozny – thank you for your invaluable contribution and insight to the Full Spectrum vs Isolate section. Dr. Magdalena Bujalska-Zadrozny has served as Deputy Dean for Science at the Faculty of Pharmacy and currently the head of Pharmacodynamics and Pathophysiology Department at Warsaw Medical University. In addition, she is the President of the Polish Pharmacological Society and a prolific author of 73 publications including works related to the endocannabinoid system. Her scientific interests are mainly related to the study of the mechanisms of pain and her research lead to patents on analgesic pharmaceutical compositions for oral administration.

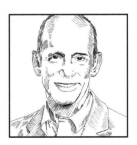

To Dr. Mercola – thank you for the tremendous work you have done and the education you have imparted to so many people regarding health and wellness issues. Your work has been honorable, insightful, and thought provoking and I am honored that you have contributed the forward to the book. Dr. Joseph Mercola, a passionate advocate of natural medicine and board certified family physician. An internationally recognized natural health expert, Dr. Mercola has achieved wide recognition through his guest appearances on leading national network shows and his multiple number one bestselling books. Dr. Mercola is also a member of the political advocacy group Association of American Physicians and Surgeons, several alternative medicine organizations.

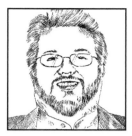

Prof. Gene Bruno – thank you for your invaluable contribution and insights to the ECS and Cancer section. Prof. Bruno has graduate degrees in both nutrition and herbal medicine and is a Professor of Nutraceutical Science at Huntington University of Health Sciences. Prof. Bruno is a well-seasoned educator for professionals, expert natural product developer, and formulator for Twinlab. A prolific author on nutrition, herbal medicine, nutraceuticals and integrative health issues in trade publications and textbooks. His latest book, co-authored with Dr. Earl Mindell, is What's in Your Blood & Why You Should Care (©2019 Square One Publishing).

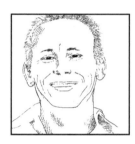

Dr. Jason Mitchell, – thank you for your contribution and insights to the ECS and Microbiome section. Dr. Mitchell is a Board Certified Naturopathic Doctor certified by the American Naturopathic Medical Certification Board (ANMCB), as well as, a member of the American Naturopathic Medical Association (ANMA). He is a natural products industry authority, expert product formulator, and primarily focused on research on nutraceuticals. He is currently the CEO and Co-Founder of Probulin,, as well as Co-Founder and President of MetaCan whose focus is on the science of nutritional endo-cannabinoid support.

Introduction

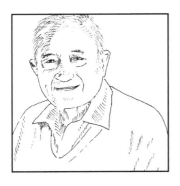

Over the last few decades research on the Endocannabinoid System (ECS) and cannabinoids has advanced through several distinct phases:

a. Research on the plant cannabinoids [mostly on tetrahydro cannabinol (THC) and cannabidiol (CBD)].

b. Research on the endogenous cannabinoids (endocannabinoids) [mostly on anandamide and 2-arachidonoyl glycerol(2-AG)].

c. Research on endogenous anandamide-like molecules.

d. Research on the underpinnings of the ECS in health and disease.

Plant Cannabinoids.

While many dozens of plant cannabinoids are known today, most research is still on THC and CBD. CBD was isolated in the late 1930's, but its structure was elucidated only in 1963. Thousands of studies have been published on plant cannabinoids and some of them are already in use as therapeutic drugs. THC has been approved as a drug (named Marinol) for enhancement of appetite, and is also used to prevent vomiting and nausea due to cancer chemotherapy. Of particular interest is CBD, which does not cause the typical cannabis psychoactivity, but is a potent anti-epileptic drug and is used in many countries in pediatric epilepsy. It is being evaluated in other therapeutic areas (graft versus host disease; schizophrenia auto-immune diseases and others). While the focus has primarily been on CBD and THC, more than 100 plant cannabinoids have been isolated from the plant. Many of these compounds have yet to be investigated for their biological activity, but initial preclinical studies show tremendous promise.

The neutral cannabinoids, such as THC, CBD, CBG, CBN, etc., are not formed as such in the plant. Typically, the cannabis plant actually synthesizes their precursors in acidic forms such as THCa acid and CBDa acid. These acids are not stable and hence their activity until recently was not investigated. However when stabilized they have shown activity in depression, suppression of nausea and anxiety.

I assume that with the legalization of medical cannabis in many countries and the passage of the Farm Bill in the US, in the near future the therapeutic use of plant phytocannabinoids will expand widely. Let's hope that this expansion will be paralleled by modern clinical trials.

Endogenous Cannabinoids.

Originally it was assumed that cannabinoids act through a nonspecific membrane-associated mechanism; however, in the 1980's the existence of binding sites in the brain was reported. Their distribution was found to be consistent with the pharmacological properties of the psychotropic cannabinoids. These binding sites are known as the CB1 receptor. A second peripheral receptor, CB2, was later identified in the spleen. Stimulation of these receptors leads mostly to protective effects.

Receptors are not present in the animal body for a plant constituent to activate it. They exist as parts of endogenous systems and are activated by compounds formed in the body. Indeed the endocannabinoid system is based on two endogenous cannabinoids, anandamide and 2-AG, which are formed when and where needed. They bind to the receptors, activate them, thus starting a reaction sequence and are then rapidly broken down by specific enzymes. The endocannabinoid system consists of the receptors, the endocannabinoids and the enzymes that build and break down these endocannabinoids. This recently identified biochemical system is of major physiological importance and is involved in many disease states, mostly as a protective entity. Indeed in many diseases an enhancement of the synthesis of endocannabinoids is noted. Such an enhancement has also been reported to occur after physical activity and may explain the euphoric feeling described after running. Surprisingly neither anandamide nor 2-AG have been administered to humans – either as drugs or for research. Are we missing something?

Endogenous Anandamide-like Constituents.
Numerous endogenous fatty acids and amino acids are present in the animal body. Hence it is not surprising that the mechanism followed for the endogenous synthesis of anandamide (which is a fatty acid bound to an amino acid derivative) will also be used by the animal body for other related compounds. Indeed there are many dozens of such endogenous compounds. We do not know all the effects they cause, but it seems reasonable to expect that many of them have physiological activity. Indeed over the last decade many such endogenous molecules have been identified to be of central importance. Thus the oleic acid amide with serine is anti-osteoporotic, the arachidonic acid amide with glycine lowers pain, the arachidonic acid amide with serine is neuroprotective, the oleic acid amide with ethanolamine helps regulate feeding. Recently it was found that the oleic acid amide with glycine has anti-addiction properties. It ameliorates the withdrawal responses in nicotine-dependent mice and opiate–dependent rats, as well as the rewarding effects of nicotine. Apparently the animal body sees addiction as a disease and as its reaction to many diseases, tries to block it. This new field of endocannabinoid research promises to yield additional, endogenous molecules of major interest. The above concise summary of cannabis research presents some of the various fields in which a large number of research groups are involved. I have no doubt that we shall continue to see major advances which will clarify many of the effects of the plant cannabinoids and the endogenous cannabinoids. And recent interest

in endogenous anandamide-like molecules may tell us something on additional ways the animal body tries to fight diseases.

The ECS As A Target In Health & Disease.
Over the past few decades, anandamide, 2-AG and several other endogenous fatty acid amides have been studied for their roles as signaling molecules involved in numerous, if not all, physiological functions in the body. Preclinical, animal and human studies support that the ECS and endocannabinoids play a key role in neurological functioning (memory, reward, mood, addiction), and governs critical metabolic processes, including regulation of blood sugar, energy production, bone building, lipid control, pain signaling, and much more. Clinically, the ECS is becoming a central target via its interactions in various neurological conditions from Alzheimer's to ALS (amyotrophic lateral sclerosis). In addition, the ECS mediates the stress response and is involved in the release of various neurotransmitters that participate in the stress HPA (hypothalamic-pituitary-adrenal axis) pathways. This specific activity provides useful insight into conditions associated with chronic stress such as anxiety, depression, inflammation, cardiovascular, gastrointestinal, skeletal involvement, and others. In summary, the ECS represents an important signaling network and orchestrates communication and connectedness throughout the entire body. While we are in the early stages of its discovery and inner workings, continued investigation and clinical trials - which are badly needed - will no doubt unravel new insights into the etiology of disease and the exciting new options for therapy. While there is an abundance of scholarly work already published, the Road To Ananda book by Carl Germano addresses many of the pertinent topics about the ECS and phytocannabinoids presented above in a simplified way to encourage further study.

Dr. Raphael Mechoulam
Hebrew University Jerusalem
School of Pharmacy
Jerusalem, Israel

THE ROAD TO ANANDA

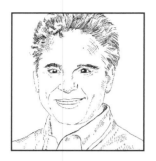

We spend much of our lives pursuing happiness and joy. From Eastern philosophies and medicine, we have learned that happiness is not brought from an external source, but rather comes from within and this internal happiness is responsible for achieving a state of bliss. In Sanskrit, this feeling of bliss is called Ananda. From an Eastern medical stance, when our mind and body are healthy and balanced, then we are able to achieve internal physiological bliss—a state referred to as homeostasis in the West. One particular modality is the attainment of homeostasis and inner bliss by balancing chakras - specific points in the body associated with different organs and system functionality. Over the past few decades, the existence of the Endocannabinoid System (ECS) as the orchestrator of homeostasis was discovered. A physiological system that strives to maintain inner balance, harmony, and peace among all organs to help attain Ananda!

The ECS is a complex network of cannabinoids we produce (endocannabinoids) and the cannabinoid receptors that accept them. Collectively, the ECS touches nearly every physiological system and orchestrates communication throughout the body. We rely on these endocannabinoids to maintain balanced health & wellness by influencing and modulating every organ including the brain, gut, bone, immune, lungs, heart, kidney, skin, etc. and their optimal functioning. The ECS synchronizes adaptation and recovery from the daily insults we are exposed to through its regulatory effects on all physiological functioning in the body. Hence, supporting and nourishing the ECS is essential to maintain inner bliss.

You likely recognize the term cannabinoid. It is the same word used to describe the active compounds found in cannabis/hemp termed phytocannabinoids as well as those pro-

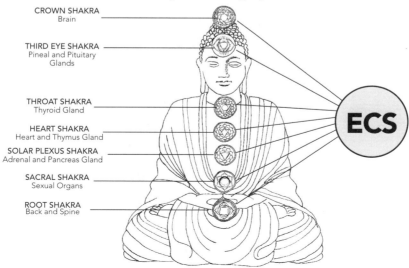

CROWN SHAKRA
Brain

THIRD EYE SHAKRA
Pineal and Pituitary Glands

THROAT SHAKRA
Thyroid Gland

HEART SHAKRA
Heart and Thymus Gland

SOLAR PLEXUS SHAKRA
Adrenal and Pancreas Gland

SACRAL SHAKRA
Sexual Organs

ROOT SHAKRA
Back and Spine

ECS

duced in the body called endocannabinoids. The words are similar because they share very similar roles in nourishing the ECS. Endocannabinoids and phytocannabinoids are so close to one another that our bodies respond similarly to the ones found in cannabis as compared to those we produce. As with any components produced in the body, at times, we don't produce enough endocannabinoids and must rely on the plant sources. Phytocannabinoids help to support our ECS to maintain optimal health and wellbeing and the most important plant source is hemp (Cannabis sativa).

While cannabis, hemp and the ECS have emerged as one of the most popular topics discussed today, their importance in health and illness will dominate medicine and nutrition for decades. The research on the ECS as a crucial modulatory system in tissues of the brain/neurological system, immune system, bone, endocrine organs, intestinal tract, etc. is remarkable. Couple this with its involvement in pathological states in the body, we are provided with a glimpse as to its compelling participation in the etiology and treatment in disease conditions. Clinicians describe both hemp phytocannabinoids and the ECS as the body's pharmaceutical treasure chest due the role phytocannabinoids play in supporting the complexities of the ECS. Nevertheless, we are in the fetal stages of research and more clinical trails are necessary.

Despite changing attitudes toward hemp/cannabis, many academic and medical institutions have been prohibited from studying cannabis and phytocannabinoids. The stigma extends beyond the plant itself and ignores the existence of a major physiological system that controls all others! This has led to a widespread dismissal or, in some cases, denial of the ECS. Due to the fundamental role the ECS plays in the body, we must dismantle the stigma attached to hemp/cannabis. To date, there are thousands of peer-reviewed published studies revealing and explaining the functional roles the ECS and as a target in the treatment of many diseases. Further, these studies validate the benefits of phytocannabinoids and how many conditions can be suitably treated by administering them. With hemp containing over 100 different phytocannabinoids, we must avoid the myopic "single magic bullet" approach by just focusing on only one - cannabidiol (CBD). The clinical efficacy of hemp is reliant on its entire family of phytocannabinoids and it is absurd to think its importance is contingent on CBD only.

Recently, we have witnessed history with the dismantling of regulations on hemp via the passage of the Farm Act 2018. It is high time that we overcome the stigma surrounding hemp/cannabis and embrace the importance this plant endows upon us. With the volume of pre-clinical and clinical research that exists, it is important for us to come to terms with the fact that our body has a major physiological cannabinoid system which is paramount to our health. With more research and clinical trials, our understanding about the ECS and the beneficial role hemp phytocannabinoids play in health and disease is paramount. Our health and pursuit of Ananda are at stake.

Carl Germano, CNS, CDN

YOUR AMAZING BODY
TRILLIONS OF PIECES, ALL INTERCONNECTED

When you marvel at the amazing intricacies of medical devices or are fascinated by the tremendous abilities of a mobile phone or computer, none compare to the human body! Made up of hundreds of tissues and organs, trillions of cells and microbes, your body is a universe of interconnected parts that all work together to keep you alive and thriving.

The relationships in your body are amazing as well. When we look at the human body, we see what appear to be separate, unconnected organ systems. Yet, from a cellular view, these organ systems reveal themselves as a single, highly organized human body. Cells, like atoms, do not work independently. They work together to create the world we know. They work together to create inner physiological peace and harmony.

Our organ systems produce messengers that speak to one another and influence each other – examples include neurotransmitters from our nervous system, immuno-transmitters from our immune system, etc. At the organ level, the hypothalamus, pituitary, and adrenal axis communicate to regulate stress response.

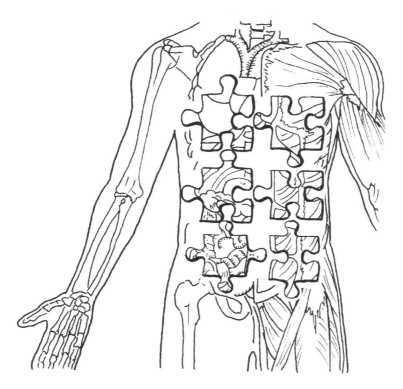

The brain, gut, and immune system communicate to maintain neurological and immune health. The liver communicates with the pancreas and circulatory system to maintain blood sugar and blood pressure. The intricate interplay of all these connections help maintain a well-balanced and healthy body. Much of this thinking is present in Eastern medical systems (Ayurvedic and Traditional Chinese Medicine), and now Western medicine is catching up to understand that our health relies on the mass communication that goes on between cells and organ systems.

As of the writing of this book, research continues to expose new connections between cells and organ systems that help build upon our understanding of the intimate link between our body and mind and its implications in health and disease. Psychoneuro-immunology, the study of the effect of the mind on health and disease, and other fields of study help us understand the connection between our thoughts and feelings and the health of our body. This broadens our understanding that our cognition is not just the brain operating independently, but rather its capacity to interact with other vital parts of our body and external influences. For example, those who practice yoga or meditate have more grey matter in their brain useful to reduce stress, anxiety, and depression.

For many, the link between body and mind is not a surprise. After all, this is essentially what Eastern medical thought has been teaching us for thousands of years. Western medicine, however, has only recently begun to understand and uncover the interconnectedness of our mind and body. Because our ECS serves as a pivotal juncture of communication and orchestration of healthy functioning in the body, it may very well be the key crossroad to the body-mind connection.

ECS

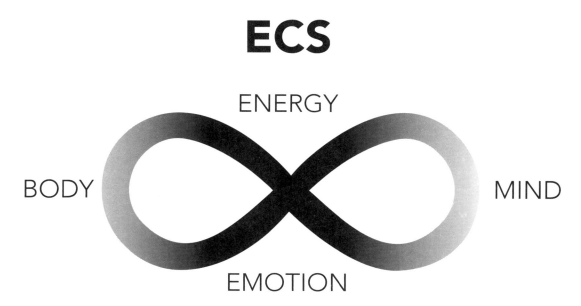

ENERGY

BODY

MIND

EMOTION

Believed to be the center of the mind and body union, the ECS is a physiological system that has evolved over the past 600 million years, but was only discovered in the 1990s. The ECS choreographs mass communication and regulatory responsibilities that solidifies vital interactions that influence the brains command over bodily functions.

Since the discovery of the ECS in the '90s, researchers have continued to uncover how it works and what effects it has on our health and wellness. We now know that the system is comprised of many receptors (endocannabinoid receptors), signaling compounds (endocannabinoids) and enzymes that control their fate. Further, these endocannabinoids and their receptors are present everywhere in the body, including the brain, heart, liver, pancreas, kidneys, lungs, skin, and reproductive tract, and affects every physiological function throughout the body.

Disrupting endocannabinoid signaling is now linked to many diseases, including neurological disorders (stress, anxiety, depression, etc.), diabetes, hypertension, liver disease, inflammatory conditions, bone health, insomnia, digestion, and many more. Over the past few decades, researchers have compiled data on the complexities of the ECS and detailed how it regulates and interacts by communicating with our organ systems. The amount of information we have on the ECS continues to grow at a rapid pace. All this research strongly indicates that the ECS is central to maintaining health and wellbeing. Through the ECS and its vital relationship with all physiological functioning, we now can understand how to maintain balance within the body and modulate it for the treatment of many degenerative diseases. The ECS is, in many ways, an adaptogenic system and a key to homeostasis in order to attain the state of bodily bliss and well-being.

",,, Modulating endocannabinoid activity may have therapeutic potential in almost all diseases affecting humans, including metabolic syndrome, diabetes, neurodegenerative, inflammatory, cardiovascular, liver, gastrointestinal, skin diseases, pain, psychiatric disorders, cancer, among others."

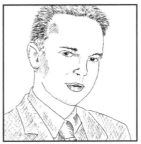
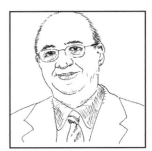

Pal Pacher   *George Kunos*

Laboratory of Physiologic Studies
National Institutes of Health, Bethesda, MD

THE MISSING PHYSIOLOGICAL SYSTEM

Do you remember studying the physiological systems in the human body in school? We learned about the skeletal, muscular, lymphatic, respiratory, digestive, nervous, endocrine, cardiovascular, urinary, and reproductive systems. At the time, I remember being taught that these systems were separate and distinct. Each was an ecosystem in-and-of-itself. However, as we now understand, the systems of our body are not separate and independent. Instead, our body is a complex interwoven network of chemical messengers and receivers. Through its massive signaling network, the ECS is the pivotal physiological modulator that connects body and mind and provides the path to equanimity.

The 1990s were a remarkable decade of discovery for the integral parts and functions of the ECS. Researchers uncovered the existence of cannabinoids produced by our bodies (endocannabinoids), and started to understand how they communicate among cells, between organs and physiological systems in our bodies. The discovery of the ECS and its modulating effects, specifically on the brain, gut, immune system, help bridge the body and mind connection as a major medical breakthrough. When supported and cared for, the ECS can provide us with health and wellness. While, conversely, when ignored, we see the proliferation of disease and unbalanced bodily functions.

Scientists also have uncovered the presence of the ECS in other animals as well. All vertebrate species, such as fish, birds, mammals, amphibians, reptiles, and humans, share this crucial internal communication system. We have even uncovered the ECS system in invertebrate marine life. Genetically speaking, the ECS has evolved millions of years ago and most likely integral to adaptation and evolution of species.

Composed of cannabinoid receptors (doorways on the cell membrane that respond to a chemical signal) and the endocannabinoids that influence them, the ECS's primary objective is to provide a stable internal environment despite harsh conditions. Due to its ability to respond to changing environments, the ECS is considered an adaptogenic system — an essential part of life that helps the body adapt to an ever-changing external and internal environment.

Endocannabinoids are transported into cells through cannabinoid receptors and then degraded by certain enzymes called FAAH (fatty acid amide hydrolase) and MAGL (monoacylglycerol lipase). Pharmacological studies into compounds that support or

THE HUMAN BODY SYSTEMS CONNECTED BY THE ECS

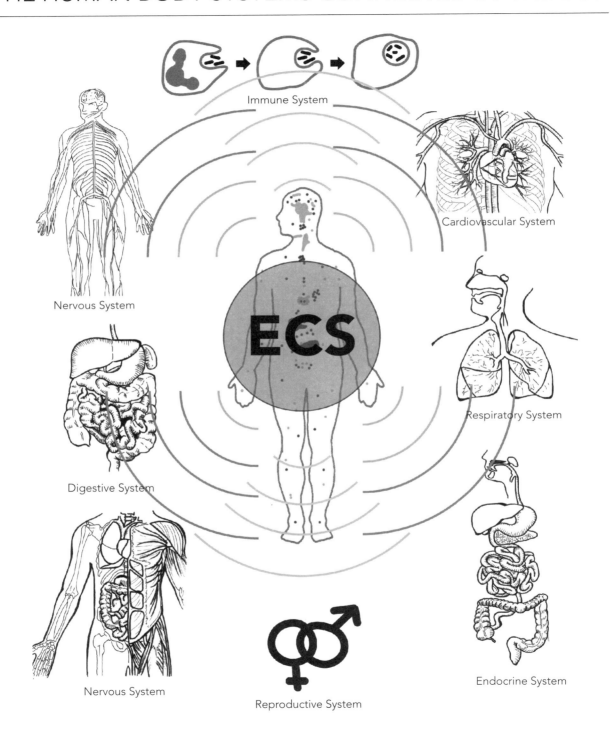

Immune System

Cardiovascular System

Nervous System

ECS

Respiratory System

Digestive System

Nervous System

Reproductive System

Endocrine System

inhibit cannabinoid receptors have provided us with valuable tools to further understand the numerous roles of the ECS. This investigation has opened up new strategies for treating pain, neurological diseases, stress/anxiety, and many other disorders.

The more we learn about the ECS, the more we understand that its discovery represents one of the most important medical breakthroughs in the history of medicine. Unfortunately, politics and stigma attached to hemp/cannabis have diverted much of the truth about the plant, as well as, research about the ECS. Unfortunately, open any physiological textbook from high school to medical school and it's very likely that you will not see anything about the ECS. For many decades, we have all been deceived about hemp/cannabis, phytocannabinoids, and the wealth of benefits they bestow on the human body. Not only have we misunderstood the cannabis plant, but there is a widespread denial of any benefits it could offer. Subsequently, the ECS had been buried since its discovery and represents a very real medical travesty. In the US, research on cannabinoids has been denied in academic and medical institutions simply because of the distorted perceptions about hemp/cannabis perpetrated by 70 years of misleading information and legal strangleholds on the plant. Fortunately, research and education is slowly disassembling this unjustified besmirchment. There has been no justification for restricting the scientific study of cannabis and the body's endocannabinoid system. This is especially true when medical researchers are discovering the undeniable benefits associated with phytocannabinoids and subsequent treatments for chronic diseases for millions of people around the world. With the recent dismantling of hemp regulations, we are now on the verge to explore and unravel the complexities of the most important botanical on the planet!

"By using a plant that has been around for thousands of years, we discovered a new physiological system of immense importance. We wouldn't have been able to get there if we had not looked at the plant (Hemp)."

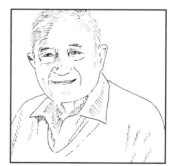

Dr. Raphael Mechoulam
Hebrew University Jerusalem
School of Pharmacy
Jerusalem, Israel

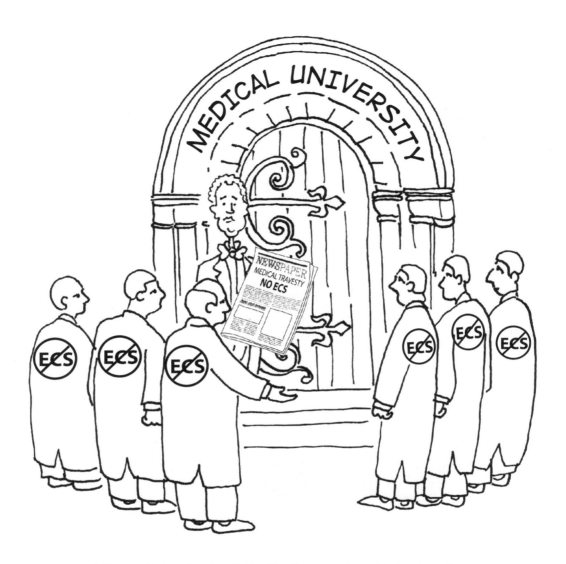

*We can't teach about the Endocannabinoid System because
non-intoxicating cannabinoids are dangerous drugs.*

In 2017, a survey by Dr. David Allen of the curriculum directors of 157 accredited American medical schools revealed that none had a department of endocannabinoid science, none of them taught the endocannabinoid science as an organized course, and only 13% of the medical schools surveyed teach the endocannabinoid science to future physicians.

http://cannabisdigest.ca/survey-endocannabinoid-system-medical-schools/

THE BRAINS BEHIND THE DISCOVERY OF ECS

As the stigma behind cannabis and cannabinoids continued to stifle research in the United States since the 1950's, Israel and Europe have been championing research that has led to both the discovery of the endocannabinoid system and a clear understanding of the tremendous influences the ECS has on the body. We now recognize its role as a master signaling control system for virtually all physiological functioning directed at establishing health, well-being, and balance — collectively known as homeostasis.

The 1960s - 1990s were a critical discovery period for the endocannabinoid system. First, in 1964, Dr. Raphael Mechoulam from the Hebrew University of Jerusalem, Israel and his colleagues isolated the psychoactive phytocannabinoid called THC (tetrahydrocannabinol). This discovery made it possible for others to understand the complexity and functionality of the endocannabinoid system further. Not long after, researchers were able to isolate and identify another dominant phytocannabinoid called cannabidiol (CBD). With both of these compounds isolated, finding the receptors that THC and CBD influence was in order.

In 1990, Lisa Matsuda announced that she and her group at the National Institute of Mental Health (NIMH) discovered a DNA sequence that encodes a receptor for THC in animals. Around the same time, Miles Herkenham and his team at NIMH mapped the locations of a cannabinoid receptor system in several animals, including humans. In 1992, at the Hebrew University in Jerusalem, Dr. Raphael Mechoulam, in collaboration with NIMH research fellows Dr. Lumir Hanus and Dr. William Devane, discovered the first cannabinoid known to be produced by the human body. They called the cannabinoid anandamide (using the prefix ananda from the Sanskrit word for bliss). The same group went on to uncover the second most important endocannabinoid since named 2-arachidonoylglycerol (2-AG), as well as other compounds that influence receptors in the body.

"... There is almost no physiological system that has been looked into in which the endocannabinoid system does not play a certain part."

Dr. Raphael Mechoulam
Hebrew University Jerusalem
School of Pharmacy
Jerusalem, Israel

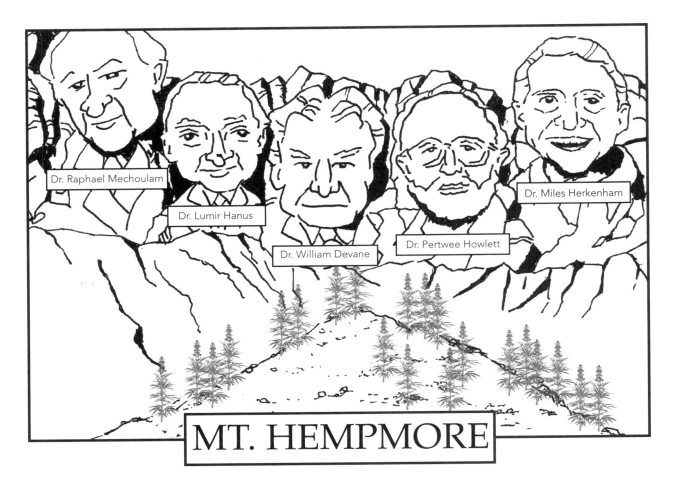

MT. HEMPMORE

After isolating THC, Dr. Mechoulam continued his work to isolate other phytoanna-binoids found in cannabis including cannabidiol (CBD). In 1986, he wrote a book called "Cannabinoids As Therapeutic Agents" describing a collection of work performed on phytocannabinoids and their physiological effects. He and his colleagues knew the profound benefits these compounds had and beneficial impact they had on the body.

After the discovery of the metabolic pathways of THC, Dr. Mechoulam and others were able to detect and unearth a major signaling network system in our body that we now call the ECS. Since this discovery, research has unraveled that the ECS helps govern neurotransmission, inflammatory cycling in the cell, pain signaling to the brain, insulin sensitivity, building bones, to name a few. In addition, studies are unfolding the usefulness of phytocannabinoids to nourish the ECS for treating many diseases including neurological (anxiety, depression, stress, PTSD, Autism, Parkinson's, Alzheimer's, etc.), inflammatory (general pain/inflammation, Irritable Bowel Syndrome, Crohn's, fibromyalgia, etc), insomnia, ocular (glaucoma, macular degeneration), bone (osteoporosis), cardiovascular conditions and diabetes.

CANNABANATOMY

While the actual biological process is much more complex and involved, essentially the ECS is a significant collection of cell receptors (endocannabinoid receptors) and compounds we produce that attach and influence those receptors (endocannabinoids). Endocannabinoid receptors can be influenced by both the cannabinoids produced by our bodies or those present in the plants we call phytocannabinoids—hemp/cannabis being the most abundant source of all.

The ECS is present throughout the entire body and plays a crucial role in governing neurotransmission and neuron communication. As such, the ECS influences numerous functions in the brain, including memory, mood, pain perception, cognition, emotions, motor function, reward, and anti-inflammatory effects. Signals from the ECS help manage the mechanisms for brain development and protection.

Today, we understand that the ECS receptors are found outside of the nervous system as well. In fact, they are present all over the body, in the intestinal tract, liver, heart, immune system, the skin, and all other organs orchestrating mass communication. In doing so, the ECS regulates a wide range of physiological effects, while always striving to maintain health and homeostasis.

As of this writing, two receptors have been discovered and thoroughly reviewed in the literature, and a third one is about to make its debut. The first is called CB1 (cannabinoid receptor 1) and the second is named CB2 (cannabinoid receptor 2). These receptors are known as G-protein coupled receptors or GPCR receptors. GPCR receptors are the most diverse group of receptors found on the cell surface and are vital for information delivery into the cell. Specifically, the cannabinoid receptors act as radars that pick up biochemical signals from every organ of the body to communicate on the cellular level. The most responsive chemical compounds to these receptors are the endocannabinoids, first discovered by Dr. Mechoulam and further research and discovery by others.

The two endocannabinoids discoverd are known as anandamide (Ananda is the Sanskrit word meaning bliss) and 2-AG (2-arachidonoylglycerol). There is new evidence that a possible third CB receptor exists (CB3) and, while it has not been named yet, it is identified as GPCR55. The initial doctrine that CB1 receptors are only found in the nervous system and CB2 receptors in immune system has now been dismantled. Research now shows that both receptors are abundant in all organ systems and play important regulatory roles either in unison or in opposing ways.

Our body's endocannabinoids (anandamide, 2-AG) are made from lipids and are taken up and broken down rapidly by enzymes in the cell. The most notorious enzymes that break down our endocannabinoids are known as FAAH (fatty acid amide hydrolase) and MAGL (monoacylglycerol lipase). The FAAH enzyme degrades anandamide, and the MAGL enzymes degrade 2-AG. Unfortunately, degradation of our endocannabinoids is rapid, and we may not be able to produce sufficient amounts leaving us in a state of deficiency. Endocannabinoids are conditionally essential for our bodies to maintain balance and prevent or treat specific medical conditions. Moreover, there is a need to use diet and supplementation to help the body receive the cannabinoids it requires and the most important source is from hemp. Hemp not only provides the dominant phytocannabinoid called cannabidiol (CBD), but also supplies a multitude of other important phytocannabinoids that participate in the benefits hemp provides the human body.

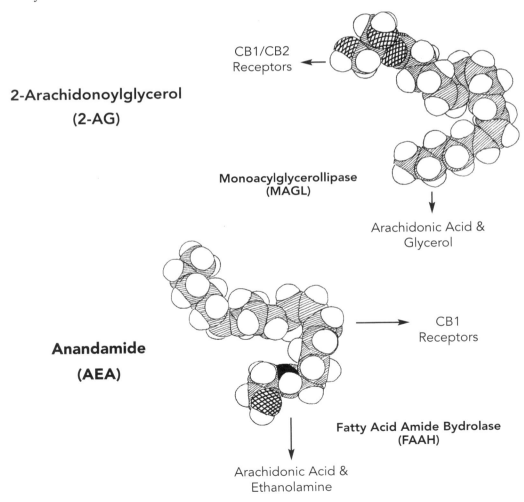

CB1/CB2 Receptors

2-Arachidonoylglycerol (2-AG)

Monoacylglycerollipase (MAGL)

Arachidonic Acid & Glycerol

CB1 Receptors

Anandamide (AEA)

Fatty Acid Amide Bydrolase (FAAH)

Arachidonic Acid & Ethanolamine

13

One way to achieve this is by consuming full spectrum CO2 extracted hemp oil from aerial parts — the richest source of phytocannabinoids. While the hemp plant contains over 100+ different phytocannabinoids, full spectrum hemp oils are the most effective as they contain the full family of phytocannabinoids - not just CBD! The collective of phytocannabinoids has been shown to be more clinically beneficial as compared to single magic bullet CBD isolates. In addition to hemp, phytocannabinoids can be found in foods such as carrots, chocolate, echinacea, clove, pepper, thyme, hops, rosemary, and other plants/herbs. Unfortunately, one would have to consume an enormous amount of these foods and spices to have any beneficial effect, as they contain only trace amounts. Hemp is really the most obvious choice for phytocannabinoid consumption and ECS support. In addition, several papers have pointed to diet, synergistic supplements, massage, acupuncture, and other lifestyle modifications as a way to support and care for your body's ECS.

SOME IMPORTANT PHYTOCANNABINOIDS IN HEMP

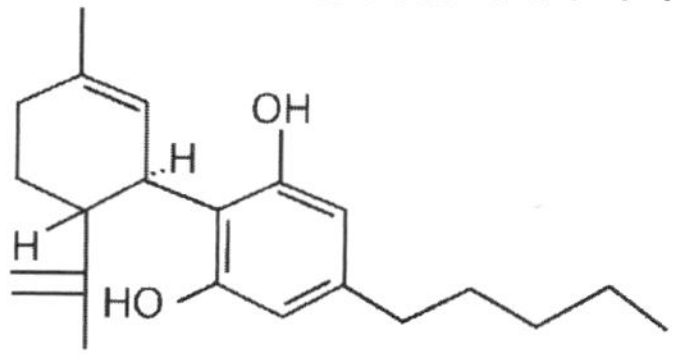

Cannabidiol
(CBD)

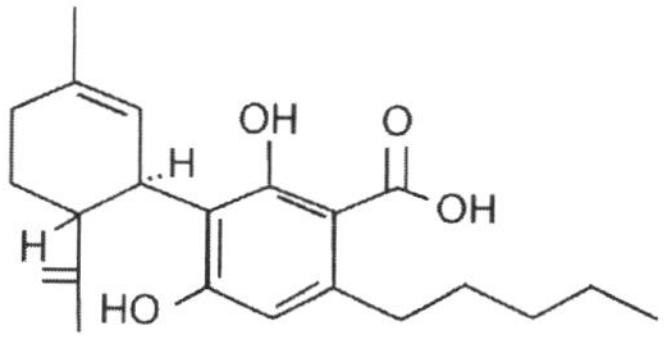

Cannabidiolic Acid
(CBDA)

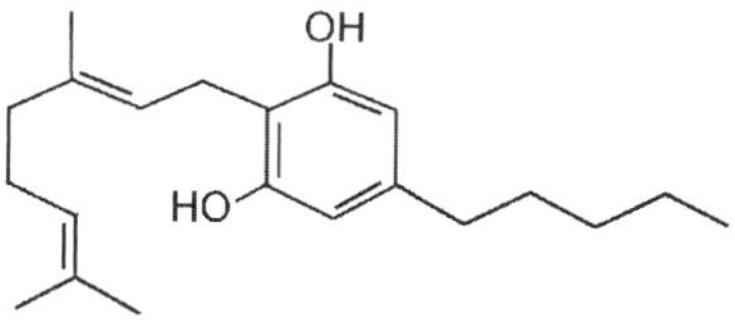

Cannabigerol
(CBG)

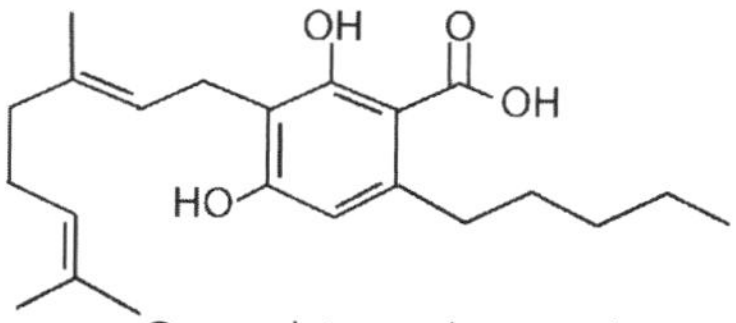

Cannabigerolic Acid
(CBGA)

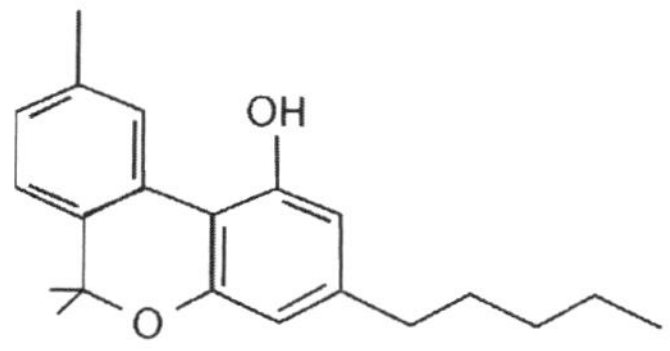

Cannabinol
(CBN)

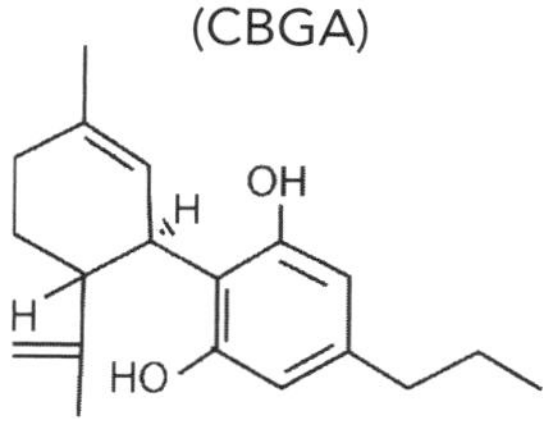

Cannabidivarin
(CBDV)

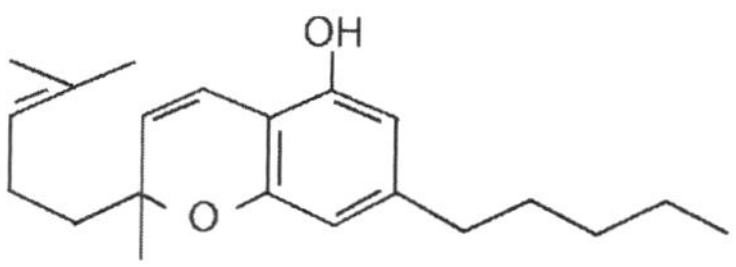

Cannabichromene
(CBC)

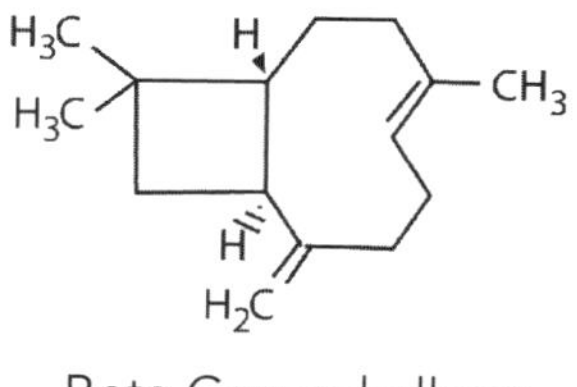

Beta Caryophyllene

ENDOCANNABINOID RECEPTOR LOCATIONS

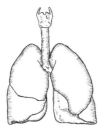

Lungs CB1- CB2

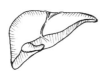

Liver CB1-CB2

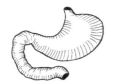

Stomach CB1-CB2

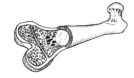

Bone Marrow CB1-CB2

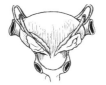

Bladder CB1-CB2

Skin CB1-CB2

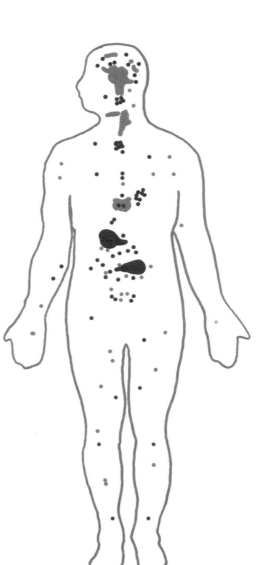

Brain CB1-CB2

Heart CB1-CB2

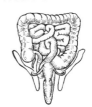

Intestines CB1-CB2

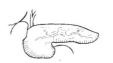

Pancreas CB1-CB2

Spleen CB1-CB2

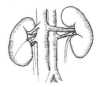

Kidneys CB1-CB2

ENDOCANNABINOIDS & THEIR RECEPTORS

The presence of endocannabinoids in our bodies is abundant and overwhelming. Researchers find more endocannabinoid receptors than the neurotransmitter receptors of serotonin and dopamine. In total, the number of endocannabinoid receptors in the body is believed to be greater than all other neurotransmitter receptors combined.

Receptors are proteins that act as doorways on the surface of cells for messengers to deliver information into the cell. They act as the cell's eyes and ears for what is happening in the body. Every cell in every organ has specialized receptors to react to signaling throughout the body. Compounds that have the ability to sit at the doorway to deliver messages into the cell are called ligands. Typical ligands you may be familiar with are neurotransmitters and hormones that bind to receptors to initiate certain and specific activity.

Endocannabinoid receptors (cannabinoid receptor 1 (CB1) and cannabinoid receptor 2 (CB2) live on the surface of cells and act as the binding sites for the endocannabinoids we produce in the body (anandamide, 2-AG). They are also influenced directly and indirectly by many plant cannabinoids (phytocannabinoids) we consume. Hemp extracts represent an important and highly concentrated source of phytocannabinoids. The most popular and dominant phytocannabinoid in hemp is called cannabidiol or CBD. However, CBD is only one of 100+ phytocannabinoids present in hemp that are equally important or more effective than CBD in addressing certain conditions. Most notably, the phytocannabinoids CBG (cannabigerol), CBC (cannabichromene), CBN (cannabinol), and BCP (beta caryophyllene - a CB2 agonist) are but a few up and coming ones that are equally important to consume with CBD.

When bound to CB receptors, cannabinoids influence numerous physiological and biochemical functions in the body. Like a scattered array of stars across a night's sky, the CB1 and CB2 receptors spread throughout the body, in all our organs and tissues. And like an individual planet with a gravitational force, they use a variety of methods to attract compounds that will alter their effects. From a genetic point of view, both CB1 and CB2 receptors share approximately half of their amino acid composition which is responsible for their identification and the amino acid sequence of both are similar. To no surprise, both CB1 ad CB2 receptors are influenced by similar cannabinoids.

•CB1 receptors are abundant in the brain, especially in the cerebellum, basal ganglia, hippocampus, amygdala, hypothalamus and spinal cord regions. They play significant roles in regulating pain signaling, memory processing, movement, motor control, and many other neurological functions. In addition to their concentration in the brain, CB1 receptors reside in the cardiovascular, digestive tract, heart, liver, lungs, immune system as well as other parts of the body. Their presence in these regions expands their activity to include functional roles in bone, heart, liver and immune modulation.

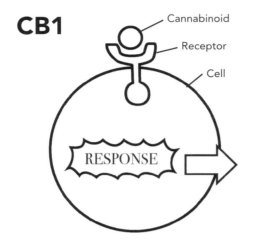

CB1

Cannabinoid

Receptor

Cell

RESPONSE

Regulating neuron development, pain signaling, learning & memory processing, movement, motor control, inflammation, bone mass, and many other functions.

•CB2 receptors are predominant in the brain and immune system, but are present throughout the entire body. Researchers have also found an abundant amount of CB2 receptors scattered throughout the brain in greater numbers along with its CB1 counterpart. In addition, CB2 receptors are present in our bones, as well as peripheral organs such as the spleen, liver, and pancreas. As situated in these organ systems, CB2 receptors have many roles, including immune modulation, bone mass enhancement, brain protection, pain and inflammation control, liver support and healthy stress response.

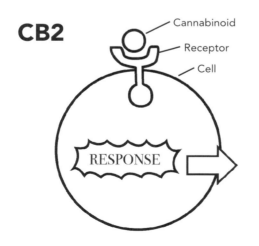

CB2

Cannabinoid

Receptor

Cell

RESPONSE

Immune modulation & autoimmunity, enhancing bone mass, protecting the brain, pain and inflammation, liver support, and healthy stress response.

As you can see, the interactions of endocannabinoids and their receptors are critical for many physiological functions in our bodies. When either endocannabinoids or phyto-cannabinoids activate CB receptors, vital communication occurs within the cell, which results in major functional effects. Interestingly, our endocannabinoids work very differently than other transmitters in the body.

For example, brain cells (neurons) communicate with each other and the rest of the body by sending chemical "messages" (neurotransmitters). These messages tell the body how to regulate certain physiological functions, as well as influencing our thoughts and emotions. Typically, neurons (a presynaptic cell) release neurotransmitters that then travel across a small gap (called a synapse) and attach to specific receptors located on a nearby neuron (postsynaptic cell). This stimulates the receiving neuron into action, triggering a set of events that allows the message to be passed along.

RETROGRADE NEUROTRANSMITTER

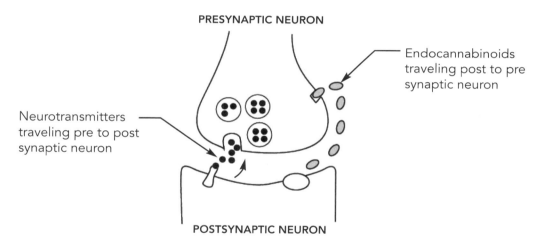

PRESYNAPTIC NEURON

Endocannabinoids traveling post to pre synaptic neuron

Neurotransmitters traveling pre to post synaptic neuron

POSTSYNAPTIC NEURON

Our endocannabinoids work in the opposite direction. By traveling from the postsynaptic neuron back to the presynaptic neuron, they exert regulatory functions by telling the presynaptic neurons to slow things down. Essentially the ECS and its endocannabinoids enable the postsynaptic neurons to reduce any neurotransmitter errors and regulates the output of neurotransmitter release. This is particularly useful in inhibiting pain pathway signaling and over stimulation in the brain. Regulating and adding efficiency in neurotransmission is part of the ECS's regulatory role to maintain balance in the body. Controlling neurons is how the ECS creates homeostasis in the body. In addition, the ECS in the nervous system is involved in neuropretection, modulating pain signaling, regulation of motor activity, building new brain cells (neurogenesis), synaptic plasticity and the control of certain phases of memory processing. Regulating and adding efficiency in neurotransmission is part of the ECS's regulatory role to maintain balance in the body. Controlling neurons is how the ECS creates homeostasis in the body.

GOING BEYOND CB1 & CB2
ADDITIONAL TARGETS

With ECS research steadily increasing and validating its major responsibility as a regulator for most physiological functions in the body, we now understand that its ubiquitous role is due to the promiscuous activity of endocannabinoids and phytocannabinoids (plant cannabinoids) beyond the CB1 & CB2 receptors. Knowing that the ECS targets all organs and influences most physiological activity, it should be no surprise that cannabinoids bind to other receptors that control critical functionality all over the body. In the past 5 years, researchers discovered several other receptors that are the target of both endocannabinoids and phytocannabinoids. Further, we've uncovered how their pervasive influences result in providing neuroprotective, anti-inflammatory, analgesic, cardiovascular, bone, eye and GI supportive effects. In studies with animals with genetically removed CB1 and CB2 receptors, endocannabinoids and phytocannabinoids continue to function in many areas. This revelation led to the discovery of how cannabinoids have an affinity to other targeted receptors in the body responsible for many central physiological activities and that endocannabinoids bind to many receptors that are not part of the endocannabinoid system.

PROMISCUOUS CANNABINOIDS

Initial research worked to define the efforts of anandamide and 2-AG that speak with the CB1 & CB2 receptors present on cell membranes - known as G protein-coupled receptors (GPCR). As a group, there are over 1,000 GPCRs that respond to other substances exerting a varied range of activities. We know endocannabinoids and phytocannabinoids can influence many of these GPCRs including:

- Anandamide activates GPCR18 which is found throughout the cerebellum, spinal cord, lungs, immune cells, small intestine, thymus and testis. This receptor influences our immune system and can lower blood pressure.

- Both anandamide and 2-AG can activate GPCR55 which is found in throughout the central nervous system, kidneys, lung, gut, liver and adrenal glands. This receptor influences pain signaling & inflammation, energy intake, lowers blood pressure, bone remodeling, and protects the brain.

- Both anandamide and 2-AG have a small effect on GPCR119 which is found in the GI tract and pancreas. This receptor effects our appetite, weight and helps regulate blood sugar.

ANANDAMIDE

RESPONSE

GPCR18
- Regulates Immunity
- Lowers Blood Pressure

ANANDAMIDE 2-AG

RESPONSE

GPCR55
- Pain
- Inflammation
- Energy
- Bone
- Brain

ANANDAMIDE 2-AG

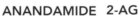

RESPONSE

GPCR119
- Appetite
- Weight
- Blood Sugar

TARGETING MORE THAN JUST CB1 & CB2

Over years of research, it is now evident that both endocannabinoids have an array of functions. This is due to their ability to seek and influence cellular targets, even those not known as GPCR endocannabinoid receptors. Some of the most influential non-CB receptors that endocannabinoids exert their effects on include serotonin receptors, peroxisome proliferator-activated receptors (PPARS), glycine receptors (GLYRS), GABA (gamma amino butyric acid) receptors, and vanilloid receptors (TRPVS).

At a glance:

- Vanilloid receptor TRPV1 (Transient receptor potential vanilloid 1) - found in high levels in the central nervous system. TRPV1 senses tissue damage and communicates potential issues with the brain. Anandamide can activate the TRPV1 receptor which is involved in the etiology of chronic pain and inflammatory conditions.

- Peroxisome proliferator-activated receptors (PPARS) - expressed all over the body, both anandamide and 2-AG help to activate PPARa, PPARg, and PPARy. When triggered, these receptors help regulate cell growth & proliferation and are involved in reducing pain & inflammation, and protecting the brain, gut, and heart.

- Glycine receptors (GLYRS) - widely expressed in the central nervous system and help to control the excitability in the brain and spinal cord pivotal for motor control and sensory processing. Both anandamide and 2-AG have been shown to influence GLYR receptors.

- GABAA receptors - a major inhibitory neurotransmitter in the central nervous system. 2-AG has been shown to potentiate GABAA receptors which are responsible for sedative, muscle relaxing, anticonvulsant and anti-anxiety effects in the body.

- Serotonin receptor 5-HT3 (5-hydroxytryptamine) - found in many areas of the central nervous system. Anandamide can bind and inactivate certain 5-HT3 activity that is involved in emesis (vomiting) and analgesic effects in the body.

TARGETING MORE THAN JUST
CB1 & CB2 RECEPTORS

TRPV1

Chronic pain and
inflammatory conditions

5-HT3

Emesis (vomiting) and anagesic
effects in the body

PPARS

Reducing pain & inflammation,
and protecting the brain, gut
and heart

GLYRS

Both anandamide and
2-AG have been shown to
influence GLYR receptors

GABA

Sedative, muscle relaxing,
anti-convulsant and
antianxiety effects in the body

ANANDAMIDE
MORE THAN JUST BLISS

Anandamide, appropriately termed the bliss molecule, attaches to the CB1 receptor, the same receptor in the brain to which the psychoactive cannabinoid THC attaches and exerts its consciousness expanding effects. While not as potent as THC, Anandamide (N-arachidonoyl ethanolamine) is appropriately viewed as a sought after molecule that has positive effects on our mood, feelings and perceptions. However, through further research, we now know anandamide also attaches to CB2 receptors and serves many other vital functions.

Neurologically speaking, anandamide is a neurotransmitter that helps produce new nerve cells, reduces inflammation in the brain, and regulates functions that produce memory, creative thought processes, reward and motivation processes, control of movement in the body, emotion response and many other functions.

In its ability to form new brain cells, anandamide acts as a mood elevator and stabilizer, useful in the treatment of anxiety and mood disorders, such as depression. Aside from its benefits in the brain, research has unraveled numerous other positive effects anandamide has on the body including balancing hormones, reproduction, and reducing pain. Anandamide also helps control cell proliferation, survival, and programmed cell death (apoptosis), which gives it a key role in the prevention and treatment of certain cancers. In animal studies, upregulating anandamide or decreasing its degradation has been shown to be useful in decreasing cancer proliferation by triggering enhanced cancer cell death.

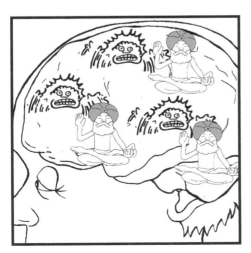

Anandamide

- **Pain Relief** - analgesic effects of anandamide are related to the TRPV-1 receptors it modulates.

- **Reward** - anandamide signaling in the reward pathway of the brain results in positive feelings.

- **Runner's High** – anandamide levels are significantly increased after exercise and tied into endorphin and opioid receptors.

- **Mood** - anandamide helps reverse symptoms of depression in animals and has been shown to be depressed in humans with stress induced anxiety.

- **Cell Regulation** - anandamide plays important roles in differentiation and development of brain cells

Additionally, some of the effects of anandamide are independent of binding to CB1 or CB2 receptors as we have seen it influences or attaches to other important receptors including the PPARs (involved in memory, learning, anti-inflammatory, lowers lipids and blood sugar), TRPV1 (involved with analgesic effects, pain signaling, bone health), GPCR55 (cannabinoid receptor that plays a role in cancer and pain), and GPCR119 (cannabinoid receptor that plays a role diabetes, insulin resistance).

So, with anandamide in our brain, why aren't we blissful all day long? First of all, anandamide is not as potent as THC in exerting psychoactive effects in the brain. Also, our endocannabinoids are synthesized and released on demand as the body needs them. Their levels are kept in check by certain enzymes that break them down, leaving us, at times, with less than desireable anemic levels. Its dismantling is caused by the enzyme FAAH (fatty acid amide hydrolase). FAAH enzymes break down endocannabinoids at a very rapid pace. When levels of endocannabinoids get too low, Endocannabinoid Deficiency states occur, which are associated with several conditions including anxiety, fibromyalgia, migraines, irritable bowel syndrome, and other inflammatory and neurological conditions.

How, then, do we keep anandamide levels high if they are known to be low? The best way is to supplement with hemp derived full spectrum cannabidiol (CBD) supplements. CBD is known to interfere with the FAAH enzyme that degrades anandamide and therefore keeps levels high (endocannabinoid tone).

FAAH ENZYME DEGRADES ANANDAMIDE

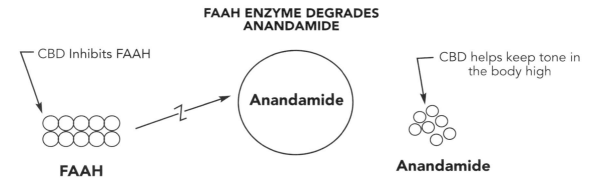

We can also add in some dark chocolate since it contains anandamide related compounds that also inhibit anandamide destruction in the brain. These dark chocolate derived compounds (N-oleoylethanolamide and N-linoleoylethanolamide) also act as cannabinoid mimics and can have both direct and indirect effects on cannabinoid receptors in the body. Truffles and kaempferol (a flavonoid found in apples, tomatoes, broccoli) also inhibit FAAH, but large quantities would be needed and clinical work needs to be done to determine an effect in the human body.

2-AG: THE WORK HORSE

Arachidonoylglycerol (2-AG) was the endocannabinoid to be discovered after anandamide. Like Anandamide, 2-AG is a neurotransmitter that attaches to both CB1 and CB2 receptors. However, 2-AG acts as a full CB2 agonist and exhibits a variety of activities throughout the body. Its unique molecular structure is responsible for many of 2-AG's biological activity. Based on the results of several structure activity relationship studies, 2-AG is a physiologically essential molecule. This appears to be the case because the CB1 and the CB2 receptors are primarily 2-AG receptors. 2-AG is the most prevalent endocannabinoid ligand (molecule that binds to a receptor) in the brain and throughout the body where it helps to regulate immune function, pain management and potentially as an inhibitor to certain types of cancer as well. Of note, levels of 2-AG in the brain are approximately 170 times higher than those of anandamide!

When 2-AG activates CB1 And CB2 receptors, many physiological processes are influenced including immunity, reduction of inflammation, insulin sensitivity, motor activity memory & learning, neuroprotection, pain signaling, mood, stress, anxiety, to name a few. Research shows that 2-AG acts as a messenger molecule that regulates the transmission of signals across brain cells and helps modulate inflammation by decreasing the inflammatory cyclooxygenase (COX)-2 enzyme in the brain (protects neurons) and throughout the body. Studies have also demonstrated that 2-AG helps minimize the spread and further infiltration of certain cancer cells as well.

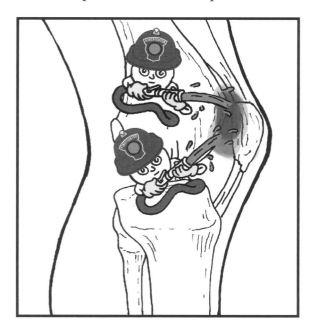

Preclinical trials show that activation of the CB2 receptor (function of 2-AG) results in reductions in pro-inflammatory cytokines (inflammatory components from the immune system) and useful in the treatment of inflammatory conditions such as arthritis, osteoarthritis, inflammation in the lung and brain, as well as inflammatory conditions in skin (psoriasis, eczema, dermatitis)

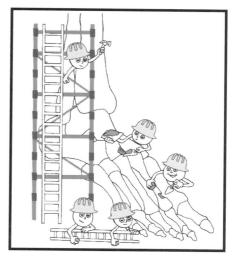

Studies in animals and humans show that activation of CB2 receptors by 2-AG in bones results in inhibiting the formation of the cells that break down bone (osteoclasts) while favoring the production of the cells that build up bone (osteoblasts)

Recently, 2-AG has been shown to potentiate GABA receptors known to inhibit excitatory behavior in the brain and are the target of many tranquilizer medications. Stimulating the GABA receptor provides for 2-AG's role in reducing stress and anxiety, inhibiting motor activity, and having sedative and muscle relaxation attributes. In addition, 2-AG also has been implicated in influencing the proliferator–activated receptors (PPAR) (involved in memory, learning, anti-inflammatory, lowers lipids and blood sugar). As we have seen with both anandamide and 2-AG, endocannabinoids do not only regulate and target the CB1 and CB2 receptors. Instead, they exert their ability to maintain health, well-being, and balance in the body (homeostasis) by orchestrating their influence with multiple receptor targets in the body that control numerous physiological effects.

Like anandamide, 2-AG is susceptible to degradation primarily by a different enzyme in the body called MAGL (monoacylglycerol lipase). The 2-AG breakdown is more complicated with at least seven other different enzymes involved in converting it back into its components, arachidonic acid and glycerol, or turning it into other active signaling molecules. An active component of Boswellia called b-amyrin has been shown to inhibit MAGL which can result in increasing 2-AG tone.

MAGL ENZYME DEGRADES 2-AG

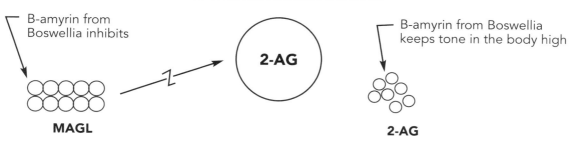

THE SEAT OF CONSCIOUSNESS:
THE ROLE OF THE ECS

What is consciousness? We all experience it, but it is hard to understand or explain. From a classical viewpoint, consciousness is defined as the awareness of everything going on around us at any given moment of time. This awareness affects our behavior, thoughts, feelings, sensations, etc. How awareness happens has been a puzzle for many years, but science has helped us unlock many of the secrets of the brain and its inner workings.

We now know that within our brains are billions of neurons interacting with each other providing vital information about how to observe or respond to internal and external stimuli. Awareness, as viewed as consciousness, occurs as an adaptive mechanism that enables organisms to react appropriately to various physical and environmental signals. This processing helps govern our very being and affects our emotions, mood, thoughts, etc. So, from a neuroscientist's point of view, consciousness is produced by the communication in our brain cells that are responsible for producing our memories, perceptions and awareness.

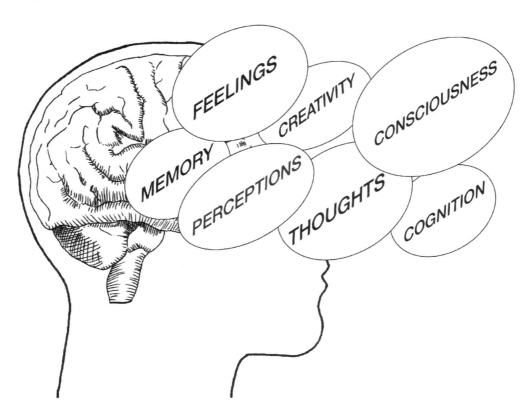

Sigmund Freud stated that daily thoughts and experiences influence our dream content suggesting that dreams were produced by the subconscious. The ECS controls various functions and neurobiological activity associated with consciousness, including mood, memory, perception, learning, cognition, reward, pain, etc., the sleep-wake cycle is yet another one. Animal studies have shown that blocking CB1 receptors or inhibiting the FAAH enzyme that degrades anandamide encourages a wakeful state. Researchers go further, hypothesizing that the ECS modulates dreams. An emotional part of sleep involves dreaming and the ECS influences our emotional states as well. They believe the ECS controls aspects of dreams by influencing and responding to our emotions, perceptions, and interactions. Post-traumatic stress disorder (PTSD) is characterized as an anxiety disorder exacerbated by recurring traumatic dreams and nightmares. Patients with PTSD have been shown to have depressed endocannabinoid levels in both hair and blood. Interestingly, research shows reduced levels of both 2-AG and anandamide promote aversive emotional memories in PTSD patients. In early Post Traumatic Stress Disorder studies, administration of cannabinoids may significantly decrease symptoms. While further clinical trials are in order, this initial work is very promising.

PARTS OF THE BRAIN AFFECTED BY CANNABINOIDS

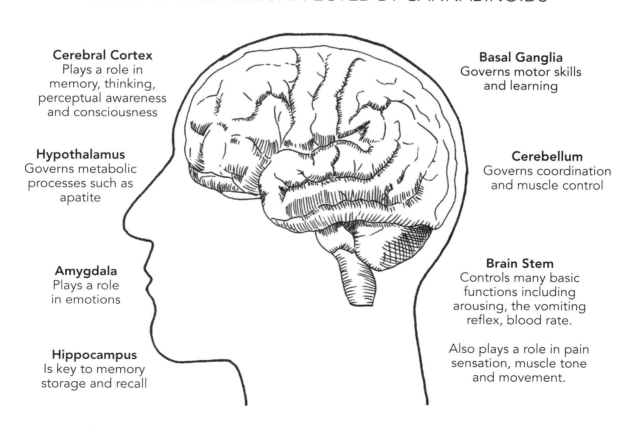

Cerebral Cortex
Plays a role in memory, thinking, perceptual awareness and consciousness

Hypothalamus
Governs metabolic processes such as apatite

Amygdala
Plays a role in emotions

Hippocampus
Is key to memory storage and recall

Basal Ganglia
Governs motor skills and learning

Cerebellum
Governs coordination and muscle control

Brain Stem
Controls many basic functions including arousing, the vomiting reflex, blood rate.

Also plays a role in pain sensation, muscle tone and movement.

A key to understanding consciousness is being further explored in modern medicine. Scientists are using anesthesia to block consciousness and investigate how and when coming into arousal—a conscious state – the various pathways in the brain control consciousness. Anesthetics can hamper communication pathways in parts of the brain and block the ability to assimilate information as compared to awake states. Therefore, arousal after anesthesia is viewed as a useful tool to study the brains mechanisms that control consciousness. Animal studies have demonstrated that the ECS is involved in circumventing the effects of anesthesia. When chemicals were used to block ECS signaling in the brain, mice were able to come out of their anesthetic state rapidly and researchers were able to map the pathways responsible for this effect.

So, in addition to regulating internal physiological processes, our ECS plays a major role in our relationship with the external environment that forms our perceptions, thoughts, emotions, etc. Through its involvement in the growth of new brain cells and forming new connections between neurons, the ECS influences our mindfulness and helps to reformat old behavior influenced by our past experiences.

Every conscious thought, perception or feeling, and everything we think or do is influenced in one or more ways by the ECS and the level of endocannabinoids! In subtle ways, the ECS is responsible for things that determine if you are thinking clearly, our personality traits, focus, being laid back & relaxed, anxiety, etc. Because the ECS can regulate key aspects of our consciousness, it also able to influence who we are, what we feel, and how we think. In many ways, the ECS is an internal reflection of you!

"It's becoming clear the endocannabinoid system plays a crucial role in the human body's inner workings. As such, a better understanding of this system — and of cannabinoids in general — will likely lead to better health outcomes."

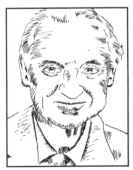

Dr. Lumir Hanus
Hebrew University Jerusalem
School of Pharmacy
Jerusalem, Israel

THE GUT, BRAIN, IMMUNE & ENDOCANNABINOID SYSTEM

Did you ever have a "GUT feeling"? It may be more than just a saying. The interplay between your GUT (intestinal tract), brain, and immune system has been the focus of many researchers over the past few decades. In my very first book published in 1997, The Brain Wellness Plan, Dr. Lombard and I wrote an entire chapter on the brain-GUT-immune connection knowing of its crucial importance to maintain a healthy brain and body. This important discovery was involved the inner workings of the intimate tridirectional communication between these three organ systems. This work has led to new fields of study including the brain-GUT connection and psychoneuroimmunology which links both physical and mental health!

Through a collection of chemical messengers from each organ, neurotransmitters from the brain and immunotransmitters from the immune system forge this intimate communication pathway. New research has further solidified the relationship as scientists now know of the existence of a lymphatic system in the brain. The lymphatic system, composed of tissues and organs, helps detoxify the body and transports white blood cells and other immune cells throughout our body. The lymphatic system is also found in regions of the brain. So where does the GUT come into play?

To complete this triad of organ system communication, we first need to transcend the traditional thinking of the digestive system as just an organ of digestion. Interestingly, your brain and GUT develop from the same tissue during fetal development and are both connected by the vagus nerve. We know that in addition to its important role in digestion, the GUT is lined with hundreds of millions of immune cells and represents our largest immune organ in the body. In addition to 70% of our immune system located in the GUT, research also tells us that the intestinal tract has over 100 million neurons (brain cells). That's right, the brain and immune system are found within the intestinal tract. So, the next time you think about the GUT as only an organ of digestion, think again! The wiring and interactions between the GUT, brain, and immune system are extremely influential in many functions and aspects of our health. Addressing gut health is more than just solving digestion issues, it can help in the treatment of neurological conditions like anxiety and depression, and even help with Alzheimer' and Autism.

The intestinal tract (GUT) encounters the most offensive agents that can harm the body, and therefore, it should be of no surprise that it is the largest immune organ in the body. Seeing as our intestinal tract is lined with neurons and immune cells that communicate with our

TRI–DIRECTIONAL COMMUNICATION

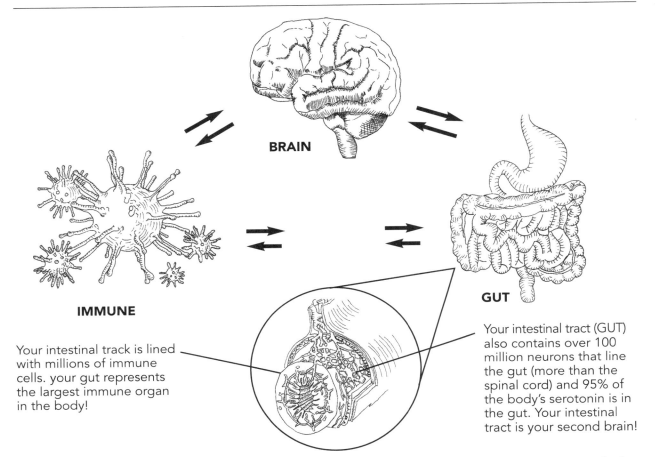

BRAIN

IMMUNE

GUT

Your intestinal track is lined with millions of immune cells. your gut represents the largest immune organ in the body!

Your intestinal tract (GUT) also contains over 100 million neurons that line the gut (more than the spinal cord) and 95% of the body's serotonin is in the gut. Your intestinal tract is your second brain!

brain and immune systems and understanding the interplay of every organ system with the ECS, the connection between these three organ systems and the ECS is complete. Both CB1 and CB2 receptors are present and very active throughout the intestinal tract performing a variety of functions equally crucial to support the GUT, brain, and immune system connection.

With the ECS widely distributed throughout intestinal tract, we can see how its effects would be significant. Research shows that the ECS helps to regulate the healthy, normal movement (intestinal motility), control of nausea and vomiting, essential to our in-stinctual feelings (GUT feelings), and "quells the intestinal fire" associated with and implicated in the etiology of many intestinal inflammatory maladies - from irritable bowel syndrome to Crohn's disease.

The intestinal immune system is constantly exposed to toxins, pathogens and allergic substances we ingest daily and must respond effectively to maintain health. The brain and nervous system's role is to sense any issues and recruit the ECS to maintain the immunes system's tolerance and response to the potential harmful environment in the GUT.

Essentially, the ECS plays a role in maintaining intestinal balance and stability (homeostasis) even when faced with both external & internal challenges to which it is exposed. While the GUT, brain, and immune system has numerous functional roles with the ECS, studies show the endocannabinoid anandamide promotes the production of macrophages, an important immune cell found in the intestinal tract. Macrophages are essential for maintaining homeostasis, this is because they help the intestinal tract fight toxins and help modulate inflammation.

GUT–BRAIN–IMMUNE–ECS CONNECTION

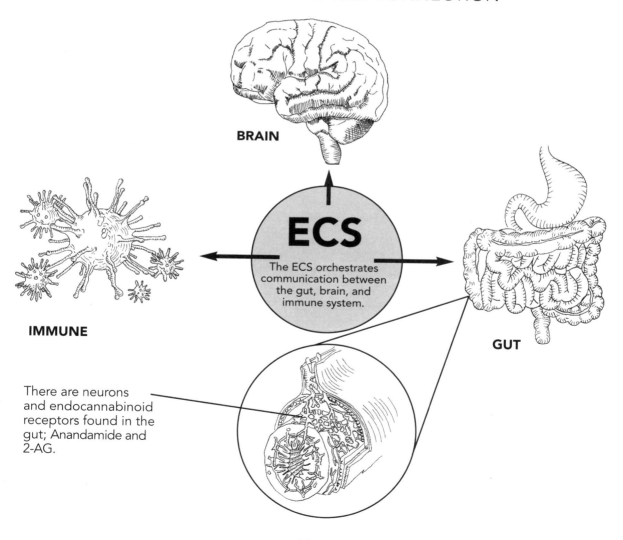

BRAIN

ECS

The ECS orchestrates communication between the gut, brain, and immune system.

IMMUNE

GUT

There are neurons and endocannabinoid receptors found in the gut; Anandamide and 2-AG.

The communication between the GUT, brain, immune system and the ECS is vital and its importance cannot be overstated. As clinical trials commence, their relationship should be a target in the prevention and treatment of many intestinal diseases. Pre-clinical studies have revealed the following focal roles of the ECS on the GUT, brain, and immune system connection including:

- The ECS helps to regulate gastrointestinal motility (rhythmic contractions), control of nausea and intestinal inflammation, and is pivotal in reducing the activity of HPA pathway, an action which helps relieve stress and anxiety

- Anandamide helps maintain immunological health in the intestinal tract, as the ECS regulates inflammation and its negative effects on GUT permeability (leaky GUT)

- The ECS controls gastric secretions/contractility, vagal neurotransmission (connection between the brain and GUT), hunger signaling and assists in proper response to foreign antigens

- Results uncover a major conversation between the immune & nervous systems with the ECS and probiotics in your intestinal tract - the endocannabidiome meets the microbiome!

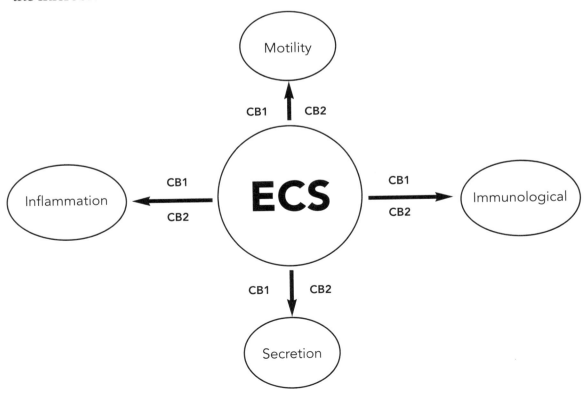

ENDOCANNABINOID SYSTEM & EXERCISE

Today, the neurological mechanisms for the beneficial effects of exercise reveal a major contributory role of our ECS. The psychological rewards associated with strenuous activity correlate well with the reported increases of endocannabinoids as a response to sustained exercise. When activated, our ECS also participates in the analgesia, reduced anxiety and feeling of well-being linked to regular exercise. Exercise is also very beneficial to the body, that is known to most everyone. Even moderate exercise over extended periods can improve your immune response, cardiovascular health, mood, and other important physiological attributes. In general, regular exercise boosts the immune system, can lowers risk of upper respiratory infections and protects against inflammation and inflammatory processes. The anti-inflammatory effects of exercise are important for a variety of reasons, from prevention of injury and reducing infections to slowing the breakdown of muscle after activity.

BENEFITS OF EXERCISE

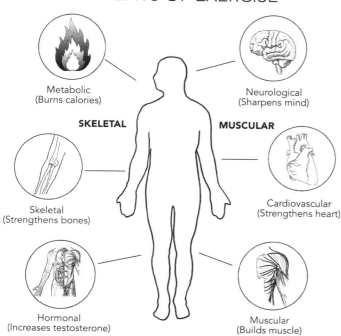

Metabolic
(Burns calories)

Neurological
(Sharpens mind)

SKELETAL　　**MUSCULAR**

Skeletal
(Strengthens bones)

Cardiovascular
(Strengthens heart)

Hormonal
(Increases testosterone)

Muscular
(Builds muscle)

At its most basic level, the function of the immune system is to protect us from the harmful effects of noxious agents like bacteria, viruses, environmental contaminants and a whole host of toxic products we deal with from exposure to various stressors on a day to day basis. Research tells us consistent activity encourages the immune system to work more efficiently for longer periods of time – the key here is moderate exercise. But too much strenuous exercise without proper recovery can be harmful by increasing oxidative stress, inflammation, muscle breakdown, and immune suppression.

Yes, there is such a thing as too much exercise! Every time the body is exposed to strenuous activity, the body handles it as if it were similar to the stress of an illness at the cellular level. Knowing the endocannabinoid system (ECS) is the key modulator of inflammation and stress and strives to adapt and maintain homeostasis, addressing its support is paramount in helping athletes and weekend-warriors recover and perform better.

Every individual, regardless of age or lifestyle has some degree of physical stress. Too much physical stress, at once or compounded, can have a negative impact on their health. Intense exercise represents one of the greatest sources of physical stress that athletes deliberately subject themselves to it on a regular basis. When your body responds to physical stress it can increase your metabolism, heart rate, blood pressure, oxygen consumption and therefore expose you to an increased free radical generation. Evidence of initial damage to muscle fibers can be seen within a short period of time after activity. Over-training and restrictive eating can also lead to reduced immune function, fatigue, increased risk of injury, and inflammation. This damage can initiate a cascade of inflammatory markers and oxidative stress from excess free radicals that both contribute to further harm to your body and negatively affects your training efforts.

The damage caused by strenuous activity has been documented in several studies where oxidative stress markers are elevated following strenuous exercise. At times, the excess free radical production causes an imbalance that can exceed the body's antioxidant defense systems, leaving an athlete vulnerable to tissue and muscle breakdown, muscle soreness, fatigue and inflammation. While muscles respond positively to exercise-induced free radicals (i.e., increasing the production of cellular antioxidants), they inevitably attack and ruin cellular structures (i.e., oxidative stress). The degree of oxidative stress is dependent on the body's ability to maintain effective antioxidant defense in response to the free radical oxidants produced from exercise. If intensity, frequency and duration of exercise exceeds the body's capacity to launch an effective antioxidant response, your body begins to show signs of an overwhelmed defense system. The results are an increase in fatigue and tissue destruction caused by free radicals.

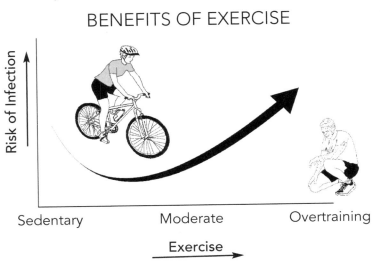

BENEFITS OF EXERCISE

Risk of Infection

Sedentary   Moderate   Overtraining

Exercise

At the microscopic level, free radicals cause lesions in integral DNA, enzymes, cell membrane lipid structures inside muscle cells that can result in cell death and intense soreness. Growing evidence exists that demonstrates how the ECS regulates free radical generation and removal mechanisms in the cell. In-vitro studies indicate that the delicate balance between free radical production and their removal by antioxidants is largely governed by the ECS. In addition, preclinical studies show that certain phytocannabinoids such as CBD act as potent antioxidants in the brain and throughout the body.

The aspect of proper recovery cannot be overstated. Recovery in any training program is important, as it assists the body to efficiently adapt to the stress caused by exercise. Recovery also allows the body to replenish energy stores, repair damaged tissues, and reduce pain and inflammation. With the immune system and stress hormones contributing to circulating inflammatory components, the damage done by inflammation is not just the overt redness, pain, heat and swelling you see in injury. Those menacing inflammatory molecules cause a reduction in joint function, as well a breakdown of muscle. When chronically elevated from strenuous activity, blood vessels dilate in muscles and joints, which causes more heat, redness and swelling. More than the swelling and heat, pain is the red flag that tells you the joint or muscle tissue is injured and inflamed.

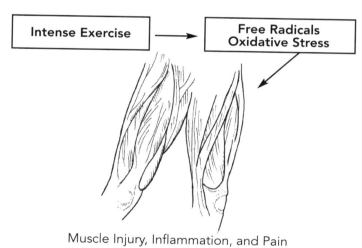

Intense Exercise → Free Radicals Oxidative Stress

Muscle Injury, Inflammation, and Pain

CB1 receptors are scattered throughout the pain processing parts of the brain and spinal cord. This tells us that anandamide and 2-AG likely play a crucial role in pain control after exercise. Studies demonstrate how the ECS participate in various physiological effects in response to exercise. These effects include vasodilation and bronchodilation required to deliver much needed blood, nutrients, and oxygen to muscles. In addition, the ECS helps regulate body temperature, motor control, energy production and aerobic capacity.

The ECS, as previously discussed, has noticeable benefits when properly nourished and supported. Exercise can help keep your ECS in shape as well. To achieve exercise induced benefits from the ECS, research reveals moderate exercise is best. Human studies reveal that the activation of the ECS results in elevated anandamide (sometimes 2-AG) levels that enhances endocannabinoid communication (signaling) throughout the body. This is beneficial because anandamide acts on sensory fibers to relieve pain.

Both preclinical and human studies support the role of CB1 activation blocking the sensation of pain in the pain sensory neurons and show increases in both anandamide and 2-AG. In human studies, reductions in pressure-pain threshold after exercise is associated with increases in anandamide and 2-AG. In addition, animal studies have revealed that exercise engenders changes in endocannabinoid pain signaling to the brain and reductions in inflammatory markers as well. In addition, elevated inflammation and oxidative stress takes its toll on the ability for athletes to maintain adequate energy production in the form of adenosine triphosphate (ATP) that can have a significant impact on performance.

ANANDAMIDE LEVELS SIGNIFICANTLY RISE AFTER ACTIVITY

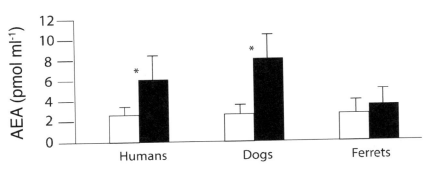

David A. Raichlen et al. J Exp Biol 2012;215:1331-1336

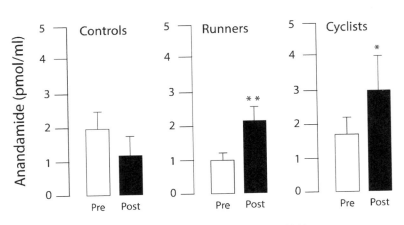

Sparling PB, et al., Neuroreport. 2003 Dec 2;14(17):2209-11

In order to manufacture energy in muscle, we must first convert the energy (calories) we consume through diet to a usable form for the body. Inside every cell lies the ability to convert the energy derived from food into a special chemical energy molecule called adenosine triphosphate (ATP). ATP serves as the currency for all energy needs.

Regardless of the type of exercise you are engaging in, whether strength or endurance, the ability to perform is based upon adequate and efficient production of ATP. Muscles depend on a constant and consistent supply of ATP produced in the part of the cell called the mitochondria. Think of mitochondria and ATP as a battery inside your cell. When it is fully charged, the cell is able to run effectively and efficiently.

The ECS also has a relationship with ATP. CB1 receptors are found in large numbers within the mitochondria as well on its surface. The presence of CB1 helps assist in regulating cell activity. In low stress conditions, our endocannabinoids stimulate mitochondrial activity, while high stress conditions our endocannabinoids regulate stress and buffer against further damage. The higher the intensity of activity, the more the muscle depends on available stores of ATP. Unfortunately, the mitochondria are an easy target for free radicals. This is because mitochondria consume most of the oxygen taken in by the cell. During strenuous activity, the more oxygen you take in, the more free radicals are produced (oxidative stress). Add in poor antioxidant defenses and you have a lethal mix resulting in damage or apoptosis of the mitochondria.

Fortunately, as we have discussed, exercise allows the body to adapt and respond to this onslaught of free radicals. By increasing antioxidant defense, the ECS orchestrates protection and regulation within the cell. The effectiveness of this adaptation depends on the health and support of the ECS as well as your training protocol, diet and supplement regimen, and adequate rest.

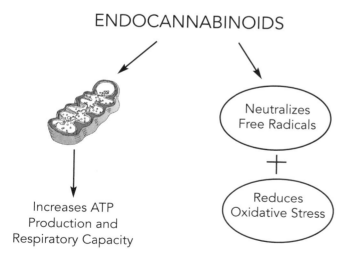

ENDOCANNABINOIDS

Increases ATP Production and Respiratory Capacity

Neutralizes Free Radicals

+

Reduces Oxidative Stress

As we have seen, our ECS is responsible for a variety of important bodily functions. It has a major influence on immune regulation, cognition, memory, anxiety, movement, sensory, neuroendocrine release, insulin resistance, eye and bone health, and anti-inflammatory effects.

The list goes on. And as mentioned earlier, the ECS is also responsible for "the runner's high." For decades, human studies have described the analgesic pain-relieving effects and emotional rewards after moderate aerobic and resistance exercise. While exercise provides both physiological and psychological remunerations, the euphoric and palliative effects are not just from the elevation of endorphins in the body.

The traditional viewpoint that exercise incites the endorphin systems responsible for the "runners high" has now been challenged by the data on the ECS's involvement. After strenuous activity, activation of the opioid and endorphin receptors as participants in pain relief has been well studied and accepted as primary evidence. Today, this has been challenged to favor the role of the ECS and its influence on both endorphin and opioid receptors. Researchers believe our endocannabinoids also play a major role in engendering mood elevating rewards, and helps you relax by reducing pain and anxiety, modulates body temperature, hormone production, and blood pressure. By inhibiting excitatory motor behavior and bringing on a sense of calm, the ECS puts the body at rest.

In human studies, both endorphins and anandamide levels significantly increase after exercise. Consequently, both CB1 and CB2 receptors are activated by exercise. The significant increase in anandamide and 2-AG levels after exercise is directly associated with reductions in pain and the euphoric feelings. This effect is partially due to our opioid system's ability to raise endocannabinoid levels after activity. Because higher levels of endocannabinoids and more stimulation of their receptors, the relief from pain and a feeling of euphoria is felt.

Exercise has also been a subject of investigation to explain the cognitive benefits achieved in both young and older adults. One mechanism that may explain this phenomenon is that elevated ECS activity also influences Brain Derived Neurotrophic Factor (BDNF) in the memory area of the brain (the hippocampus). This effect has been tested in both animal and human studies. The results showed improved memory in several preclinical trials. In the findings, researchers demonstrated how the ECS activates receptors that significantly increase our neurobiological rewards linked to strenuous exercise. The more intense the exercise, the more the ECS involvement we see. The higher anandamide levels climb, and the greater the rewards that give us the feeling of a "runner's high" with the added benefit of better memory.

No doubt, the psychological and analgesic effects of exercise are directly responsible for why many people become habitual in their exercise routines. In addition to the rewards the ECS endows upon us, our endocannabinoids also use intense activity to restore and replenish energy. For this reason, the ECS should be seen as a pivotal target of recovery for athletes.

ENDOCANNABINOID DEFICIENCY

As with many compounds we produce in the body, there are times and/or conditions where we do not produce enough, which consequently leads to deficiencies. Whether due to genetics, medications, illnesses, or aging, examples of deficient compounds (hormones, enzymes, chemical messengers, etc.) are abundant and are associated with certain diseases. For example, many neurotransmitters are associated with diseases including deficiency of acetylcholine in Alzheimer's, deficiency of dopamine in Parkinson's, and deficiency of serotonin in depression. Similarly, disturbances of the endocannabinoid system resulting in reduced levels of anandamide or 2-AG have been linked to numerous illnesses and diseases in humans.

Over the past 2 decades there has been a growing interest in certain illnesses that are associated with deficiency of endocannabinoids in the body. In animal studies where endocannabinoid deficiency was mimicked by deleting the CB1 or CB2 receptors, Alzheimer's, diabetes, stress and anxiety conditions, inflammation, and heart disease are but a few conditions associated with the deficit. In humans, reduced levels of both anandamide and 2-AG have been found in patients with post-traumatic stress disorder (PTSD), stress induced anxiety, depression, neurological and inflammatory conditions demonstrating the importance of keeping our endocannabinoid tone healthy and the potential for treatment - again, clinical trails are needed.

POTENTIAL ECS DEFICIENCY CONDITIONS

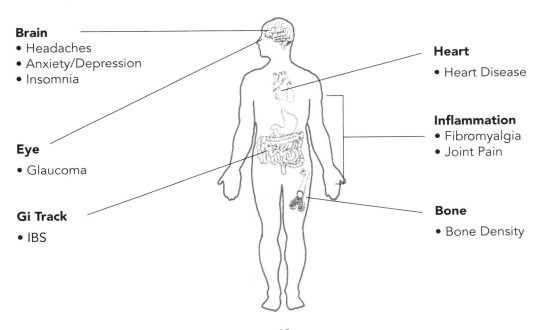

Brain
• Headaches
• Anxiety/Depression
• Insomnia

Eye
• Glaucoma

Gi Track
• IBS

Heart
• Heart Disease

Inflammation
• Fibromyalgia
• Joint Pain

Bone
• Bone Density

In 2008 and 2016, Dr. Ethan Russo published papers that helped further the term "Endocannabinoid Deficiency" (ECD) by describing how insufficient levels of endocannabinoids would adversely affect digestion, mood, anxiety, sleep, and pain and inflammation. In addition, low endocannabinoids or poor functioning of the endocannabinoid system were further associated as the cause of migraines, fibromyalgia and irritable bowel syndrome. Associations of decreased levels of endocannabinoids were revealed in the spinal fluid of migraine sufferers, multiple sclerosis patients, and reduced functioning of endocannabinoids in the spinal cord resulting in low threshold for pain as seen in fibromyalgia.

"Endocannabinoid deficiency may underlie the pathogenesis of migraine, fibromyalgia, idiopathic bowel syndrome, and numerous other painful conditions"

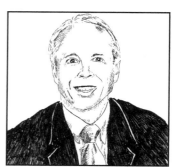

Dr. Ethan Russo
Director fo Research and Development
International Cannabis and
Cannabinoids Institute

At first glance, blocking CB1 receptors results in exaggerated responses to acute stress and produces neurological changes as seen in mood disorders including reduction in neuron development and increased levels of inflammation in the brain.

Other studies further strengthen the existence of ECD by revealing deficits in endocannabinoid production or poor signaling of the endocannabinoid system in motor coordination conditions, Alzheimer's, stress induced anxiety, diabetic nephropathy and a growing list of other conditions that can be suitably treated with phytocannabinoids. New data has unveiled the association between various psychiatric disorders (anxiety, depression, etc.) and with alterations in endocannabinoid levels as seen in animals and humans with PTSD.

In animals, promoting 2AG levels is associated with reduced anxiety and prevents stress-induced anxiety associated with anandamide deficiency. Additionally, acute 2-AG reduction increases anxiety which is normalized by increasing anandamide levels or stimulating CB1 receptors. In a way, both anandamide and 2-AG seem to serve as biological markers in blood and cerebrospinal fluid when measured and evaluated in various conditions from migraines to anxiety states. Lastly, deficiencies in the ECS are not just restricted to their classical receptors and endocannabinoids. Studies show that GPR55 (possible CB3 receptor) deficiency in animals is associated with increased obesity, reduced physical activity, and significant reductions in insulin signaling in the liver and muscle.

OMEGA 3 & YOUR ENDOCANNABINIOID SYSTEM

Understanding the global role of the Endocannabinoid System (ECS) is to maintain health, well-being and balance in the body, it is dependent on a balance of the right types of fat via diet and supplements. Since the discovery of omega 3 and omega 6 fats in the late 1920s, there has been enormous interest in how they act as precursors of many messenger molecules in the body. Several scientific studies have explored the link between omega 6 (corn, sunflower, safflower, soy, and cottonseed oils) to omega 3 (fsh oils, hemp seeds, walnuts) status and the health of the ECS. We now understand how omega 3's are involved in the production of endocannabinoids (anandamide, 2-AG), activating cannabinoid receptors in the body, as well as regulating inflammation and immunity.

While higher omega 6 to omega 3 diets are often inflammatory and have been associated with increased risk of cardiovascular disease, anxiety, depression, neurodegenerative conditions, and certain cancers, the opposite is true for high omega 3 to omega 6 diets. Scientists discovered a pathway in the body that converts omega 3 fatty acids (docosahexaenoic (DHA) and eicosapentaenoic acid (EPA)) into more potent molecules called omega 3 endocannabinoid epoxides. Studies also suggest that the anti-inflammatory effects of high omega 3 diets could be governed by the conversion of DHA and EPA into omega 3 endocannabinoids. These molecules have also been shown to help dilate blood vessels, decrease the viscosity of blood, and involved in many other physiological functions.

OMEGA 3ˢ & YOUR ENDOCANNABINOID SYSTEM

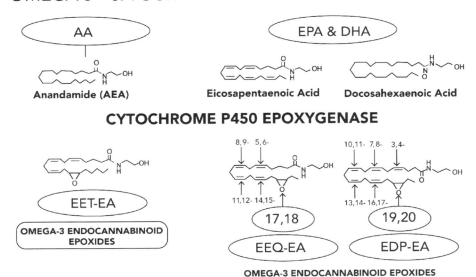

Omega-3 fatty acids are essential for both structural and functional aspects of the brain. Moreover, higher intakes of omega fatty acids DHA and EPA helps prevent or treat neurological and neurodegenerative conditions. Interestingly, inflammation is at the core of numerous diseases and involves a complex cascade of inflammatory signaling. Metabolites of omega 3's include compounds known as resolvins. The resolution of inflammation is a complex process where several key compounds are involved - omega 3 derived resolvins being some of the most important. Resolvins are responsible for expediting certain phases of inflammation in the brain, kidney, lungs and vascular system and restoring homeostasis in inflamed tissues. Both omega 3's and resolvins also reduce the inflammation involved in the promotion of certain cancers.

Because anandamide and 2-AG are produced in part from the presence of omega-3 fatty acids (and some omega 6) in the body, it is important to retain a proper balance of omega 3 to omega 6 fats. New research points to an intricate interplay between the endocannabinoid system, omega-3's and the immune system in protecting the brain and its functions. Some studies show that DHA and EPA help support neurological function, immune expression, and retinal development by influencing the gene expression of CB1 receptors. In addition, a compound called DEA (doco-sahexaenoylethanolamide) synthesized from the omega-3 DHA fatty acid is structurally similar to anandamide. The similarity between the two compounds allows it to bind to cannabinoid receptors. DEA can also stimulate the ends of neurons involved in communication (neurites) and neurotransmitter release sites (synaptogenesis), which help develop neurons in the memory section of the brain (the hippocampus). In addition, other studies reveal that EPA, but not DHA, significantly increased production of neural stem cells, which is associated with higher levels of the endocannabinoid 2-AG.

The relationship between the ECS and fats are further established by the findings that low levels of essential omega 3's are inked to pain, inflammation, anxiety, and many of the other conditions associated with endocannabinoid deficiency. Studies have revealed that omega-3 deficiency reduces endocannabinoid production and endocannabinoid receptor activity in the body. By increasing omega-3 fatty acids along with sufficient endocannabinoid tone, we may be able to offer improved treatments for migraines, fibromyalgia, irritable bowel syndrome, anxiety, inflammatory conditions, neurological conditions and overall stress challenges and consequences. Maintaining a healthier omega-3 to omega-6 ratio along with phytocannabinoid supplementation from hemp extracts may help us ward off several degenerative diseases and supports proper functioning of the ECS. If you don't get enough omega 3's, your ECS will suffer and so will you! So, omega 3 and phytocannabinoids together act like a "multi vitamin" for the ECS. Obviously, clinical trials are in order here, but preclinical data is promising.

THE ECS IN PAIN & INFLAMMATION

An estimated 1.5 billion people worldwide suffer from chronic pain–more than diabetes, heart disease and cancer combined. The sensation of pain is usually associated with stimuli resulting from certain disease conditions and/or tissue injury, however, at times, pain has no clear cause. Nevertheless, chronic pain comes with tremendous emotional and financial tolls and often presents a significant socioeconomic burden.

> ## Common Inflammatory Conditions That Can Lead To Chronic Pain
> •Arthritis •Asthma •Sprains •Carpal Tunnel Syndrome •Bursitis
> •Myositis •Fibromyalgia •Gout •Trauma •Over Training •Food •Allergies

Unfortunately, standard pain medications (opioid drugs, NSAIDS) have not provided a clear answer to treatment. For example, NSAID's (aspirin, Acetaminophen, Ibuprofen) and opioid drugs (Oxycontin, Hydrocodone, Morphine) have significant limitations, adverse effects, tolerance issues, and dependence concerns. NSAIDS also can cause erosion in the intestinal tract, impair memory, and can damage the kidney and liver. More serious consequences have been associated with opioid pain medications use and abuse. The use of opioids has grown precipitously over the past few decades reaching the magnitude of a global epidemic. Opioid abuse has multiple deleterious effects on various organs through mechanisms that are not completely understood. The current opioid epidemic is a serious public health problem, with immense individual, social, and healthcare costs. For these and many other reasons, it is imperative that we develop an anti-inflammatory lifestyle (diet, exercise, meditation, etc.) and seek healthier alternatives to deal with pain. While a significant amount of data shows acupuncture, chiropractic, yoga, herbal supplements can provide effective alternatives to standard treatment, a well-supported Endocannabinoid System is the most important part of a protocol to treat pain and inflammatory conditions.

Pain is the most common manifestation of both acute and chronic inflammation. The brain and immune system are both involved with the sensation, cause and perception of pain and the inflammatory response is intimately tied into your immune response. For instance, when an injury is sustained, any microbe that enters the body elicits an immediate immune response which includes the release of a variety of pro-inflammatory chemicals (chemokines, interleukins, etc) that not only cause inflammation but are integral in causing pain. Interestingly, when an injury or inflammation is present, there is an abrupt rise in the level of anandamide and 2-AG in efforts to control the response to the injury or inflammatory process. This is another example of the regulatory roll that the ECS has by modulating the inflammatory process.

It should not be of any surprise that our nervous system–brain, spinal cord, and peripheral nerves–is central in generating and stopping pain. It is the nervous system acting with the immune system that generates chemical messengers that cause pain. On the flip side when things are in balance, both organs are capable of producing chemicals that are pain killers as powerful as morphine. We can influence how much of which kind of these chemicals we make by utilizing diet, exercise, meditation, and supplements–especially hemp phytocannabinoids, such as beta caryophyllene, CBG and CBD, can support our endocannabinoid system's participation in controlling inflammation and pain.

Extracts from cannabis have been used for analgesic effects and anti-inflammatory conditions for thousands of years in Eastern medical modalities. In the U.S., cannabis was widely utilized as a patented analgesic medicine during the 19th and 20th centuries and was described in the United States Pharmacopeia. Only in recent decades have we begun to understand the specific pain relieving effects of the hemp's active phytocannabinoids via their action on the body's ECS. The endocannabinoid system is now known to be one of the key regulators in managing pain sensation and inflammation at all stages of pain processing pathways.

Before we can understand how the ECS helps manage pain, it's important to know how pain works. The sensation of pain is caused by a complex interplay of interactions between messengers (cytokines, mediators) and inflammation caused by internal or external forces. Many studies have documented the role of endocannabinoids and phytocannabinoids in influencing specialized receptors that detect harmful stimuli called nociceptors and suppressing nociceptive processing. When phytocannabinoids are administered orally, suppression in the activity of nociceptive receptors is seen in various parts of the brain and nervous system. Also, our endocannabinoids (anandamide and 2-AG) influence diverse immunological effects that are able to alter inflammation in the cell (inflammatory response) and pain signaling (nociception) to the brain. Up-regulation of CB1 and CB2 is observed in several models of pain and studies point to the anti-nociception activity when various cannabinoids are administered. Additionally, both endocannabinoids are increased following various pain conditions which further demonstrates a regulatory effect of the ECS.

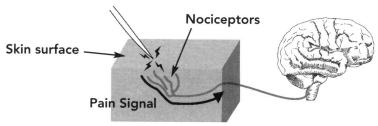

ANANDAMIDE/2AG SIGNALING

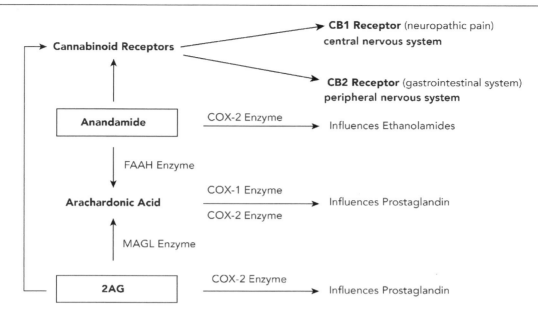

Accordingly, the ECS, endocannabinoids, and various phytocannabinoids have profound effects on controlling pain and inflammation by:
- Influencing the inflammatory cycle and response in the cell, including the eicosanoid pathways that omega 3 fish oils effect.
- Inhibiting excitatory neurotransmitters involved in pain perception.

We also are interested in the activity and contributions in specific areas of the brain with respect to pain conditions. In the limbic area of the brain, CB1 receptors help with the emotional expression of pain. In the spinal cord, CB1 receptors help regulate the transmission of pain to the brain by inhibiting neurotransmitters associated with pain sensation. In the the spinal cord, CB1 is expressed in the excitatory neurons and helps regulate the transmission of pain stimulation to the brain by blocking neurotransmitter release. In addition, CB1 receptors have analgesic effects in peripheral tissues by delaying pain signals.

In the peripheral tissue, CB2 receptors are widely located on immune cells and are a perfect target for influencing inflammatory pain processing. CB2 receptors influence inflammatory cycling related to pain by suppressing inflammatory messengers and neurotransmitters involved with pain perception. In addition, the ECS helps to regulate immune response and its ability to generate and secrete endocannabinoids and downregulate the expression of immune inflammatory factors that influence tissue inflammation.

2-AG SIGNALING IN THE BRAIN

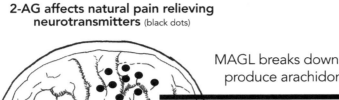

2-AG affects natural pain relieving neurotransmitters (black dots)

Arachidonic acid causes inflammation

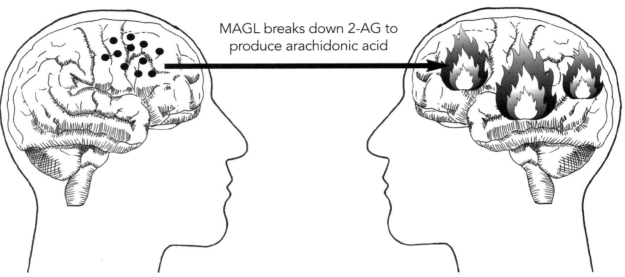

MAGL breaks down 2-AG to produce arachidonic acid

In preclinical studies, the ECS endocannabinoids block pain stimuli and the mechanisms by which anandamide and 2-AG were shown to reduce visceral sensation and pain have been revealed. In animal studies, the ECS has been shown to reduce inflammatory flare-ups, pain and joint neuropathy in models of arthritis. In patients with osteoarthritis, increased blood levels of 2-AG and an upregulation of genes expressing CB1 and CB2 associated with pain expression was noted as compared to healthy controls. Stimulation of CB2 receptors participates in anti-nociceptive signaling in neuropathic pain or inflammation by acting on immune cells as well as specialized cells in the brain. Recently, in animals, CB2 receptors were found on endorphin containing cells revealing interplay between our ECS and opioid systems. While there is strong data suggesting the therapeutic potential of endocannabinoids therapy in arthritis and chronic pain conditions, more clinical trials are needed.

Because of the ECS connection to the GUT, brain, and immune system, we can see clearly the ways in which the endocannabinoids help regulate and control intestinal inflammation. Anandamide plays a pivotal role in maintaining immunological health in the intestinal tract and regulates inflammatory pathways that disrupt digestion and absorption. At the same time, both anandamide and 2-AG help reduce inflammation in various parts of the brain and throughout the body.

The ECS also plays important roles in controlling intestinal inflammation and the link between stress and abdominal pain. It should be no surprise then that clinical studies on patients with inflammatory bowel disease enjoy positive symptomatic effects when the ECS was supported. Both pre-clinical and clinical studies have revealed the medical potential of modulating the ECS and/or utilizing phytocannabinoids in various neuro-inflammatory diseases from multiple sclerosis to dementia. In addition, evidence suggests that phytocannabinoids supporting CB1 and CB2 receptors have a neuroprotective role in brain inflammatory conditions. The take home point here is CB1 and CB2 support. Utilization of phytocannabinoids that influence or attach to both receptors is essential such as combinations of CBD and beta caryophyllene.

SYNTHESIS OF PROSTAGLANDINS

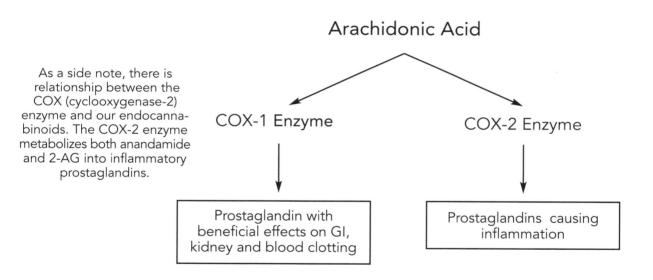

Arachidonic Acid

As a side note, there is relationship between the COX (cyclooxygenase-2) enzyme and our endocannabinoids. The COX-2 enzyme metabolizes both anandamide and 2-AG into inflammatory prostaglandins.

COX-1 Enzyme

COX-2 Enzyme

Prostaglandin with beneficial effects on GI, kidney and blood clotting

Prostaglandins causing inflammation

Lastly, studies show that endocannabinoid levels fluctuate in many inflammatory conditions including irritable bowel syndrome, migraines, fibromyalgia, brain injury, multiple sclerosis, arthritis, atherosclerosis, and many more. Due to the activity and influence of the ECS, phytocannabinoid administration is crucial in the strategy and therapeutic protocol to treating pain and inflammatory conditions. This is especially true since inflammation is at the heart and soul of all degenerative conditions and impacts several levels of disease development. In summary, preclinical and clinical studies using phytocannabinoids or by influencing endocannabinoids have been shown to provide both analgesia and anti-inflammatory effects which provides insight into promising therapeutic application for humans.

THE ECS & SLEEP

Sleep is a fundamental indicator of our well-being and we spend a third of our lives in a sleep state to accomplish the goal of maintaining good health. The National Institute of Neurological Disorders and Stroke at the National Institute of Health reports that sleep plays a housekeeping role that removes toxins in your brain that build up while you are awake as well as many other health benefits. The National Sleep Foundation, whose mission is to improve health through sleep education, evaluated the scientific literature and determined sufficient sleep requirements for all age ranges. While they vary across the lifespan, a minimum of 7 – 9 hours was determined to be adequate for most adults. Depending on what statistics you read, we unfortunately live in a "zombie nation" characterized by a majority of people who do not get adequate sleep. We pay a hefty price, in the billions, for the direct and indirect costs associated with our sleepless nation, including medical, accidents, work absenteeism, etc. A major public health problem to say the least! How we manage getting to sleep and staying in restful sleep is part of our internal biological process regulated by our endocannabinoid system where anandamide and 2-AG activate cannabinoid receptors associated with regulating sleep.

EFFECTS OF SLEEP DEPRIVATION

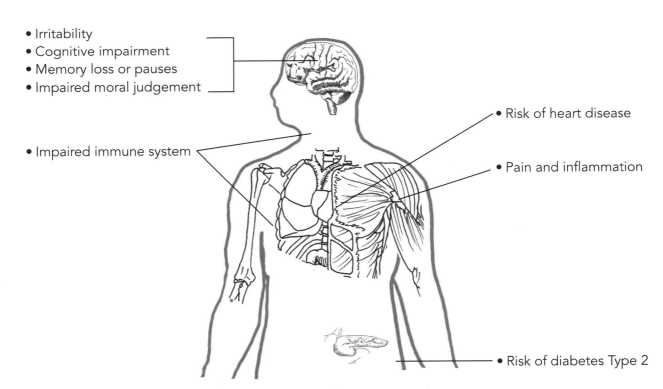

- Irritability
- Cognitive impairment
- Memory loss or pauses
- Impaired moral judgement

- Impaired immune system

- Risk of heart disease

- Pain and inflammation

- Risk of diabetes Type 2

Billions of dollars are spent on prescription sedatives, over-the-counter sleep aids, and herbal sleep supplements. With easy access to sleep aids, both prescription and over the counter, it is no wonder why many become addicted to their use. Some of the most popular prescription sleep medications, such as Ambien, Restoril, Lunesta, Sonata, among others focus on influencing the body's GABA (gamma-ami-nobutyric acid) receptors to promote sleep. GABA is a major inhibitory neurotransmitter found throughout the nervous system and is responsible for relaxation in the brain and muscles. One interesting sleep inducing dietary cannabinoid-like molecule that acts on the CB1 and GABA receptors and helps inhibit the breakdown of anandamide is the fatty acid oleamide. Oleamide is a molecule produced in the body from oleic acid as found in oilve oil. Acting as a substrate for the cannabinoid degrading FAAH enzyme, oleamide uses up FAAH, saves anandamide degradation and thereby keeping anandamide levels high. In addition, oleamide's interaction with GABA receptors produces sleepiness and promotes the healthy deep sleep cycle called REM (rapid eye movement). In preclinical studies of sleep deprivation, oleamide accumulates in the cerebrospinal fluid and helps to induce sleep by modulating benzodiazepine-sensitive GABA receptors and mimics similar cannabinoid behavioral effects of anandamide. Once activated, oleamide exhibits potent sleep inducing properties, shortens the time to induce sleep, and lengthens the time spent in one of the deepest phases of sleep.

OLEAMIDE → FAAH → OLEIC ACID

ANANDAMIDE → ARACHIDONIC ACID

Today, sleep scientists have switched focus to other neurons called orexins and their receptors. These neurons and their receptors have the ability to communicate with the endocannabinoid system. Anatomical studies reveal that endocannabinoid receptors and orexin receptors have overlapping distribution throughout the brain and have an intimate cross communication with each other. Orexins help regulate several physiological processes including the sleep/wake cycle. When our bodies have an increased activity of orexins, which promotes wakefulness and activity, and our endocannabinoids are working to inhibit excitatory behavior in the brain, then we can achieve sleep homeostasis.

Preclinical studies show that a lack of normal sleep causes dysregulation within the ECS. Because of the lack of sleep, it's important for us to support CB1 receptors, which helps us recover from interrupted sleep patterns and stabilize our sleep stages. Sleep regulation involves various parts of the brain, neurotransmitters and other messengers orchestrating proper sleep/wake cycling. Essentially, the quality and length of our sleep is influenced not only by our biological and physiological rhythms, but also by the regulatory role of our ECS. When our ECS is able to balance our biological and physiological processes, then we can achieve sleep homeostasis.

OREXIN, GABA, GLUTAMATE INTERACTION

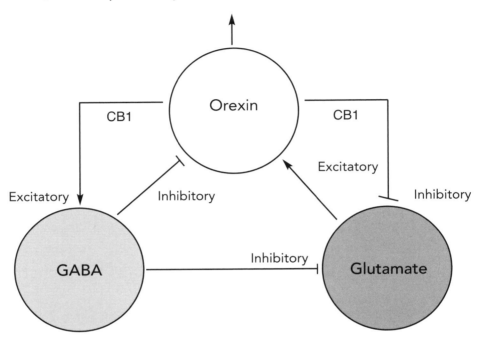

Contrary to what you may believe, sleep is an active process. In fact, many parts of the brain are just as active as when we are alert and awake. Active processes which occur during sleep deliver positive effects to our cognition, memory, immunity, blood pressure, blood sugar and many other physiological functions. What's more, these processes are regulated by our ECS. It is therefore, no wonder, that sleep deprivation increases risk of hypertension, inflammation, heart attacks, strokes, diabetes, stress, and impaired immune response – all of which are conditions that a well-balanced ECS is able to regulate.

In sleep therapy and treatment, two sleep cycles are targeted, non-rapid eye movement (NREM) and rapid eye movement (REM) sleep. NREM sleep occurs when transitioning from the wake state to the process of falling asleep, with brain wave activity slowing until the deepest delta brain wave sleep occurs. REM sleep begins 90 minutes after falling asleep and is characterized when most of our dreaming occurs. REM is also when we typically process our recent experiences. Studies show that the ECS helps regulate activity in many areas of the brain that are key for sleep cycling and our endocannabinoids have been found to act as potent sleep-inducing molecules.

STAGES OF SLEEP

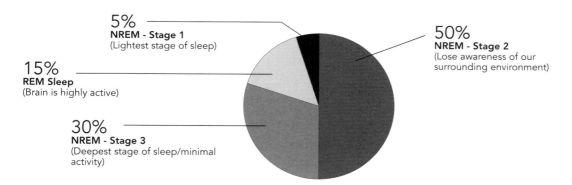

5%
NREM - Stage 1
(Lightest stage of sleep)

50%
NREM - Stage 2
(Lose awareness of our
surrounding environment)

15%
REM Sleep
(Brain is highly active)

30%
NREM - Stage 3
(Deepest stage of sleep/minimal
activity)

Both anandamide and 2-AG are located in the parts of the brain (hippocampus and hypothalamus) that control REM sleep and waking states. Pre-clinical data indicates that endocannabinoids, anandamide specifically, trigger REM sleep and both endocannabinoids influence the CB receptors that modulate sleep cycling. When the endocannabinoid CB1 receptor is chemically blocked, wakefulness is enhanced. Interfering with the transporter that takes anandamide into the cell to be degraded can also help enhance sleep.

Research continues to show that endocannabinoids are controlled by our circadian rhythm. Endocannabinoids have been shown to influence melanin-concentrating hormone (MCH), located in the hypothalamus, which promotes REM sleep and helps restore sleep in animals with insomnia. Interestingly, 2-AG plays a major role in increasing REM sleep by activating CB1 receptors that stimulate MCH. In addition to 2-AG's role, in preclinical studies, enhanced levels of anandamide in the hippocampus induces REM sleep as well. Also, 2-AG promotes sleep by making the brain more sensitive to adenosine (by product of energy metabolism)—a known suppressant of arousal wake states.

Other studies show that sleep disorders are related to a dysfunctional endocannabinoid system and an increase in activating CB1 receptors promotes sleep-inducing effects. Cannabidiol (CBD) is a phytocannabinoid that has become increasingly popular in the marketplace. This is partly because of CBD's ability to improve numerous conditions including insomnia and healthy sleep cycles. For example, in preclinical trials, CBD has been shown to increase adenosine sensitivity and helps support CB1 receptors that trigger the release of this sleep-inducing molecule. In addition, animal studies show that higher doses of CBD increase REM sleep and block anxiety induced disruption of REM sleep. In the same vein, human studies of patients with insomnia who were given higher doses of CBD saw an increase in total sleep time and a decreased arousal during the night. Through interactions and support of our cannabinoid receptors, we help the ECS function properly and regulate processes like sleep.

ECS & STRESS/ANXIETY

Illness, loss of job, divorce, medical expenses, horrible boss, bad relationship, etc. – these are some of the stressors we deal with in our lives that contribute to chronic stress, anxiety, depression and related conditions. Left unresolved, these stress situations contribute to ill health and increased risk for major degenerative diseases including cardiovascular, cancer, diabetes, neurodegenerative, and the list goes on. Exposure to chronic stress disrupts our ability to adapt physiologically and results in poor communication and function in the brain and other organ systems. While we all feel stressed from time to time, it is our ability to cope, adapt and recover in order to stay healthy. Unfortunately, chronic stress is on the rise and when our bodies are exposed to high stress levels for a prolonged period it can also lead to the development of psychological disorders (anxiety, depression, post-traumatic stress disorder) as well. As the major signaling system striving for balance and equilibrium in the body, the ECS helps us adapt to various day to day stressors and assists in recovery in all organ systems. In both animal and human studies, the endocannabinoid system has been implicated in orchestrating balance and support in the various pathways involved in the stress response and helps in calming excitatory activity in the brain that can exacerbate anxiety conditions.

STRESS EFFECTS ON MENTAL CONDITIONS

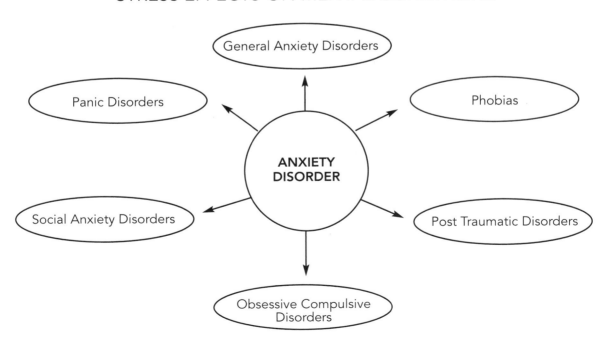

Anxiety and depression are the most common mental illnesses affecting tens of millions of adults every year. These mental states are often a reflection of an imbalanced body and mind and a disruption of homeostasis. While our stress response is a natural adaptive physiological process, chronic stress exposure sets the physiological stage for internal disruption as a contributor to the etiology of disease development. Current nutritional and mind-body intervention focuses on improving our stress resilience. If our bodies can easily and efficiently adapt to environmental, metabolic, physical, and psychological stress, then we can reduce and undo damage. Today, a large number of studies support the idea that the ECS helps regulate stress, mood and anxiety through its adaptogenic and regulatory action on various receptors and regions of the brain.

STRESS EFFECTS ON MENTAL CONDITIONS

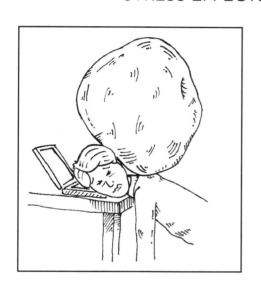

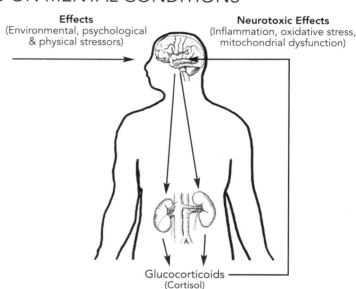

Effects
(Environmental, psychological & physical stressors)

Neurotoxic Effects
(Inflammation, oxidative stress, mitochondrial dysfunction)

Glucocorticoids
(Cortisol)

A number of preclinical studies demonstrate that the ECS helps in the management of anxiety, depression and their related behaviors by governing neurotransmission and influencing TRPV1, GABA and endocannabinoid receptors. Having counteractive activity, anandamide stimulation of CB1 receptors and blocking TRPV1 receptors results in reducing anxiety in various animal studies. While anandamide has established its role as an anti-anxiety cannabinoid, 2-AG's role has just begun to be interpreted. Preclinical studies show animals with genetic deficiencies of 2-AG induce both anxiety and depression states while increasing 2-AG reduces anxiety stress behavior. In clinical studies of patients with Post Traumatic Stress Disorder (PTSD), higher levels of CB1 receptors are found in regions of the brain associated with fear and anxiety as compared to controls. In addition, PTSD patients have significantly reduced levels of both anandamide and 2-AG. It is interesting to note that when anandamide levels are too low, the brain compensates by increasing the number of CB1 receptors since they are involved in the extinction of traumatic memories.

Interestingly, chronic stress exposure enhances the activity of FAAH which lowers anandamide levels and inhibits our capacity to adapt to daily onslaught of stressors. When stress affects the body this way, it also fosters poor neurological communication and function in the brain. As the major physiological system responsible of maintaining homeostasis, the ECS helps the body adapt to various stressors. The ECS coordinates our body's effort to diminish the effects of stress and aids recovery in the brain and other organ systems. The endocannabinoids anandamide, 2-AG, and the endocannabinoid receptors CB1 and CB2, are all expressed in key sections of the brain and other organ systems that are intimately involved in stress, anxiety, emotions, and fear.

ANANDAMIDE EFFECTS ON STRESS RESPONSES

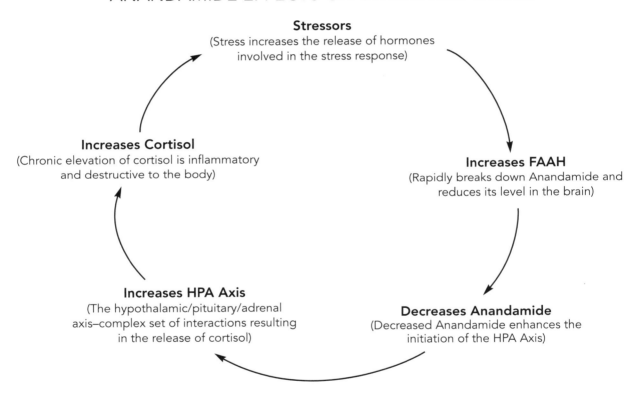

Stressors
(Stress increases the release of hormones involved in the stress response)

Increases FAAH
(Rapidly breaks down Anandamide and reduces its level in the brain)

Decreases Anandamide
(Decreased Anandamide enhances the initiation of the HPA Axis)

Increases HPA Axis
(The hypothalamic/pituitary/adrenal axis–complex set of interactions resulting in the release of cortisol)

Increases Cortisol
(Chronic elevation of cortisol is inflammatory and destructive to the body)

For instance, when CB1 signaling in the body is impaired, anxiety and poor physiological response to stress occurs. For CB1 signaling to be most efficient, our body must have an ample supply of anandamide. As mentioned previously, animal studies where the anandamide degrading fatty acid amide hydrolase (FAAH) enzyme is inhibited, a significant reduction of anxiety and mental stress was noted. Studies in humans demonstrate the same effects. Patients treated for depression show that anandamide levels in the blood correlate with significant emotional swings and stress caused a reduction in the brain's anandamide level and an increase in the stress hormone cortisol.

Essentially, concentrations of anandamide levels are negatively associated with stress conditions and decreased levels are a key biomarker to predict stress induced anxiety. Therefore, enhancing endocannabinoid tone becomes a viable strategy to treat stress, anxiety, and its related conditions. The best way to improve anandamide levels is via the consumption of full spectrum phytocannabinoid rich hemp oil standardized for its cannabidiol (CBD) content. This is because CBD is uniquely able to inhibit the rapid breakdown of anandamide by FAAH and also influences other targets of stress and anxiety. For instance, CBD inhibits adenosine uptake and 5-hydroxytryptamine 1A receptor (5-HT1A-R), as well as increasing levels of serotonin. Essentially, brain circuits involved in anxiety as well as regulatory roles in the hypothalamic-pituitary-adrenal (HPA) axis/pathway involved in our stress response, work more efficiently with an ample supply of anandamide. When our cells have a sufficient supply of both endo-cannabinoids, our bodies can more easily restore homeostasis.

The HPA axis is a term used to represent the pivotal interactions between the hypotha-lamus, pituitary and adrenal gland to help regulate the physiological response to stress in the body. Communication between the ECS and key organs involved in stress control is particularly evident within the HPA axis. This vital axis is responsible for controlling corti-sol and other stress hormones and is responsive to communication from CB1 receptors. In addition, the HPA helps regulate body temperature, circadian rhythm, metabolism, thyroid function, hormonal health, fluid regulation, and expression of cortisol.

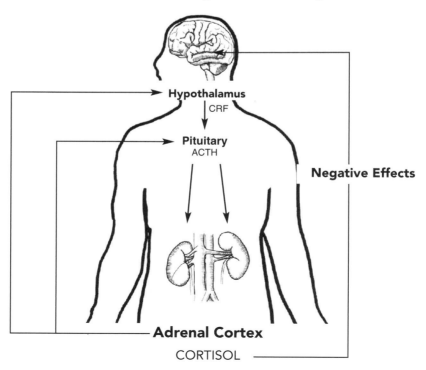

Because the HPA is responsible for cortisol levels, when overactive, it can lead to destructive imbalances in the body. A focal point of stress reduction therapy is reducing excess cortisol production from the adrenal glands to correct the dysregulation of the immune system, excess inflammation, anxiety, stress, and fatigue. Through proper production of anandamide and 2-AG and/or consumption of phytocannabinoids from full spectrum hemp we can potentially undo the effects of an overactive HPA and restore homeostasis in the body.

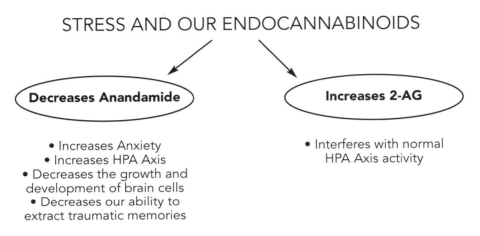

STRESS AND OUR ENDOCANNABINOIDS

Decreases Anandamide
- Increases Anxiety
- Increases HPA Axis
- Decreases the growth and development of brain cells
- Decreases our ability to extract traumatic memories

Increases 2-AG
- Interferes with normal HPA Axis activity

The relationship between anandamide and stress conditions and subsequent treatments is well understood. New data, however, is beginning to establish a role for 2-AG as well. Chronic exposure to stressors also impairs 2-AG signaling and communication in the body and reduced 2-AG levels are associated with stress conditions. Increasing 2-AG concentrations has been shown to reduce anxiety as well. In animal studies, 2-AG signaling seems to help modulate emotional behavior and lessen anxiety when exposed to stress. In addition, by decreasing the levels of monoacylglycerol lipase (MAGL), the enzyme that degrades 2-AG, reductions in the symptoms of anxiety were realized by keeping endocannabinoid tone high. In humans, alterations in the ECS are also seen in patients with clinical depression. In several studies, the connection between significantly low levels of 2-AG were observed in patients with major depressive disorders. In cardiovascular patients where we can observe reduced levels of 2-AG, it helps predict depression after heart surgery. In addition, lower 2-AG levels have also been found in patients with post-traumatic stress disorders (PTSD). The ECS is the subject of enormous attention as a target for treating stress, anxiety, depression, PTSD, and associated conditions. Clinical trails utilizing both CBD and beta caryophyllene for full CB1 and CB2 support are in order, yet current data is promising.

ECS & BONE HEALTH

With over 200 million women and men affected by osteoporosis, a condition characterized by a significant risk of fractures due to loss of bone mass and density, we need to find new ways to increase bone health. When we think of bones, we typically assume it is a stone hard substance that is firm and solid. Truth is bones are much more complex that we usually imagine. Bone tissues give our body its shape and our muscles rely on a strong hold to bones in order to put our bodies in motion. But bones are not a dead, solid object in our body. Our skeletal system is quite active and constantly changing as a means of support and protection for all of our biological functioning. Though it is strong and firm, the skeletal system is an adaptive feature of our body. In addition, studies have established the skeletal system shares a meaningful relationship with our endocannabinoid system. The ECS is not only a contributor to regulating bone mass, understanding the relationship between ECS and the skeletal system can also help us identify maladies and provide treatment of bone diseases such as osteoporosis.

OSTEOPOROSIS

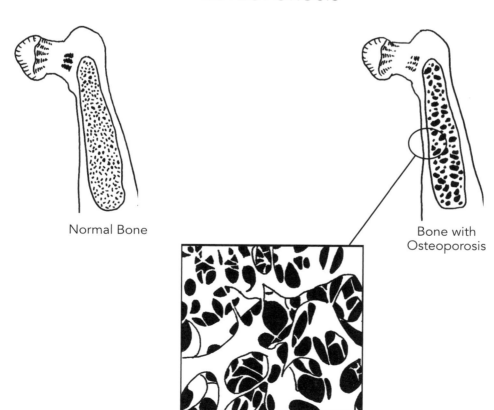

Normal Bone

Bone with
Osteoporosis

Bone is a metabolically active tissue that is continuously undergoing a process of renewal and repair known as "bone remodelling." Unfortunately, as you read this book, millions of cells known as osteoclasts are trying to break down your bones. Simultaneously, millions of cells called osteoblasts are trying to build and repair your bones. This breakdown and buildup process, referred to as remodeling, occurs throughout our entire lives. The objective is to minimize osteoclast activity (bone breakers) while supporting osteoblast activity (bone makers)—processes that go beyond supplemented calcium, magnesium, vitamin D and menaquinone-7

BONE MAINTENANCE

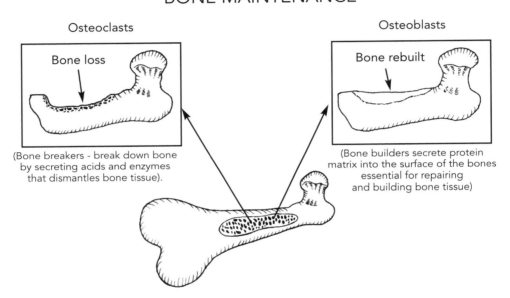

Osteoclasts

Bone loss

(Bone breakers - break down bone by secreting acids and enzymes that dismantles bone tissue).

Osteoblasts

Bone rebuilt

(Bone builders secrete protein matrix into the surface of the bones essential for repairing and building bone tissue)

Bone health is influenced by exercise, diet, inflammation, and hormones, all of which also influence the ECS. For that reason, it's no wonder the ECS plays a major role in bone physiology and homeostasis. Endocannabinoids and their receptors influence bone cell differentiation, survival and function. Both endocannabinoids, 2-AG and anandamide, and their receptors, CB1 and CB2, are present in osteoblasts and osteoclasts. In fact, the ECS is found throughout bone tissue. Research has revealed a very complex interaction between our skeleton and several organ systems, especially the central nervous system (CNS). The communication between the CNS and our bones is vital to the proper building of healthy bone tissue. In addition, preclinical studies show numerous connections between our bones and the brain—especially the brain stem, hypothalamus, and cortex. Of note, the brain to bone communication is beautifully orchestrated by our ECS. Specifically, anandamide stimulates CB1 receptors in bone, which then sends signals to suppress the release of norepinephrine—a hormone that inhibits bone formation. In animal studies, researchers tracked CB1 receptors and found that as the animal ages, the contribution of CB1 receptors to bone building benefits increased as the CB1 receptors matured.

While, activation of CB1 receptors influences brain to bone communication, our CB2 receptors are also hard at work. It is well established that 2-AG stimulation of CB2 receptors reduces both the number and activity of bone breaking osteoclasts. Studies show that activating CB2 receptors also increases bone mass by increasing the number and activity of bone building osteoblasts.

THE BRAIN/BONE CONNECTION

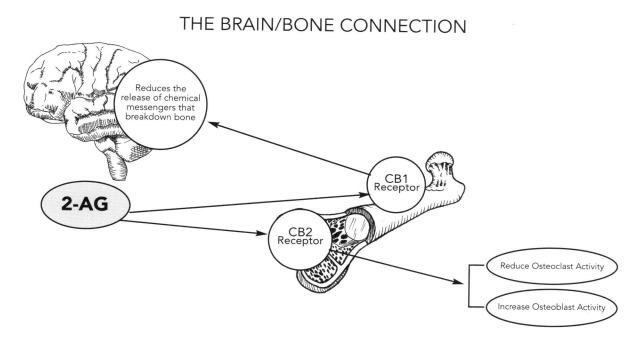

In addition to the beneficial role our endocannabinoids have on bone via CB1 and CB2 receptors, they must contend with other bone degrading receptors as well. Studies suggest that osteoporotic patients exhibit stimulated transient receptor potential vanilloid type 1 (TRPV1) stimulation and a reduction of CB2 receptors in osteoclast cells. This is not surprising, as TRVP1 is known to inhibit calcium access to skeletal tissue, which has a damaging effect on bone density. This inverse relationship of reduced CB2 receptors and elevated TRVP1 suggests a functional communication between both receptors that occurs inside osteoclasts. In studies where TRPV1 receptors are genetically deleted in animals, CB2 receptors are increased and osteoclast activity is reduced. These results demonstrate that the ECS is essential for the maintenance of normal bone mass by osteoblast and osteoclast CB2 signaling. Therefore, supporting and promoting CB2 receptor activity is a viable strategy to keep bones healthy. The phytocannabinoid beta caryophyllene, found in hemp, clove, and pepper, is a potent CB2 agonist which may prove to be a novel anti-osteoporotic therapy.

Studies into bone health and the functional role of the ECS is still in its infancy. Overall, more studies on the role of our ECS and endocannabinoid signaling in bone cells can offer further insight on harnessing the ECS's potential and therapeutic use of phytocannabinoid therapy in the treatment of bone disorders

In addition to beta caryophyllene, CBD may play an important role as well. One particular study investigated that our endocannabinoid receptors not only are involved in bone formation, but have important activities to strengthen specific tissues that connect broken bones. When CBD (with or without THC) was administered to animals, the CBD group healed faster and had stronger new bone formation.

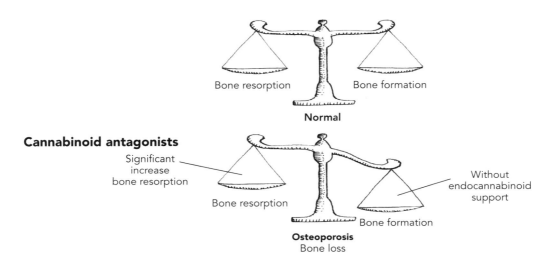

Many studies exist demonstrating the role of the endocannabinoid system as an integral player in the regulation of bone mass in health and in disease. However, many questions remain that will require clinical trials. Nevertheless, pre-clinical data shows that bone cells are abundant in CB1 and CB2 receptors and have the capability to synthesize or break down endocannabinoids. Mechanisms also need to be defined as to the whether the ECS is also influenced by typical processes involved with bone maintenance including hormonal, immune, exercise, and other factors. Basically, studies into bone health and the functional role of the ECS is still in its infancy. Overall, clinical trials are required to further describe the role of our ECS and endocannabinoid signaling in bone cells. Such information is critical and can offer further insight on harnessing the ECS's potential and therapeutic use of phytocannabinoid therapy in the treatment of bone disorders.

ECS, PHYTOCANNABINOIDS & CANCER

Cancer is a leading cause of death in the United States as well as the world, second only to heart disease. In fact, over 18 million new cancer cases have been reported worldwide as per the World Health Organisation International Agency for Research on Cancer. One in five men and one in six women worldwide, develope cancer during their lifetime. The endo-cannabinoid system (ECS), when properly maintained or utilized has tremendous potential as a prospective treatment source, for certain cancers. Medical researchers are now seeing the opportunities to use the ECS as a primary target for addressing several pathways in the development and growth of cancer.

We are now beginning to understand how phytocannabinoids (cannabinoids found in plants, such as hemp) can play a major role in influencing the ECS's involvement in cancer. This is because the ECS plays regulatory roles in inflammation, immunity, and anti-tumor activity. Supporting the ECS with phytocannabinoids can influence signaling pathways that help control tumor growth and maintenance. Today, a growing body of pre-clinical data provides further insights on the focus of the ECS and cannabinoids to target various cancers.

GLOBAL CANCER INCIDENCE

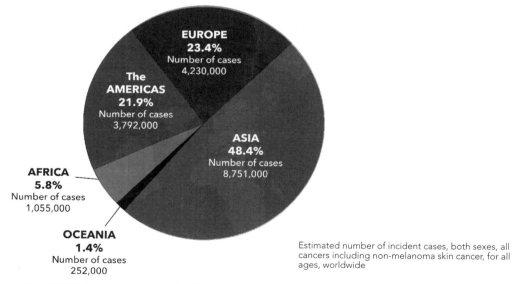

EUROPE
23.4%
Number of cases
4,230,000

The AMERICAS
21.9%
Number of cases
3,792,000

ASIA
48.4%
Number of cases
8,751,000

AFRICA
5.8%
Number of cases
1,055,000

OCEANIA
1.4%
Number of cases
252,000

Estimated number of incident cases, both sexes, all cancers including non-melanoma skin cancer, for all ages, worldwide

While the role of the ECS in cancer pathology is not entirely understood, there are clear indications of its involvement in cancer tissue activity. In preclinical cancer studies, the ECS (receptors and endocannabinoids) and phytocannabinoids were found to be involved with tumor suppressive activity by inhibiting proliferation, increasing apoptosis (cell death), and blocking angiogenesis (blood supply) to tumors. Research has also shown that phytocannabinoids have been successfully used for various purposes in cancer therapy. Initially, phytocannabinoid administration to patients have been focused on alleviating nausea, pain and to stimulate appetite. Today, scientific investigation extends their application to include anti-tumor properties, drug resistance problems during cancer treatments, and diminishing cancer treatment side-effects. Although there is a body of research on the use of psychoactive THC in the treatment of cancers (as well as the combination of THC and CBD), this discussion will be limited to the effects of non-intoxicating phytocannabinoids only.

Working within the ECS, phytocannabinoids may influence key processes that affect tumor development. Specifically, non-intoxicating phytocannabinoids, such as CBD, CBG, CBC, and CBDA, have been shown to exert anti-proliferative/pro-apoptotic effects for a variety of tumor cell lines. In other words, phytocannabinoids help reduce the growth of cancer cells and help promote their death. Researchers have noted this effect of phytocanniniods with human breast carcinoma, human prostate carcinoma, human lung carcinoma, human colorectal carcinoma, human gastric adenocarcinoma, C6 rat glioma, rat basophilic leukemia and transformed thyroid cells. In addition, different phytocannabinoids exert diverse anti-cancer activity, which speaks to the importance of utilizing full spectrum hemp derived extracts as compared to single cannabinoids, such as CBD isolates. Nevertheless, while researchers continue to investigate the anti-cancer effects of the numerous phytocannabinoids found in cannabis, CBD has the most studies published to date. Therefore, while we will discuss much of what studies have demonstrated on the effects of CBD in cancer, this is, by no means, the definitive picture of why cannabis is so important to treating and preventing cancer.

Laboratory research has demonstrated that CBD exerts anti-metastatic (i.e. reducing the spread of cancer to other organs/tissues) and pro-apoptotic effects on human glioma cells. Likewise, CBD administered to mice significantly inhibited the growth of subcutaneously implanted human glioma cells. In follow-up laboratory studies, researchers looked at the mechanisms that caused the change in cancer cells. Results revealed that CBD activated caspases (protease enzymes that play an essential role in programmed cell death). In addition, CBD was found to activate early production of reactive oxygen species (ROS) in the glioma cells, and depleted intra-cellular glutathione—although CBD did not impair non-cancerous glia cells. In other words, the CBD directly influences the body's ability to hinder cancer growth.

CBD's antitumor mechanism was also investigated in human lung cancer cells. Results showed that in response to CBD tumor cell lines exhibited increased levels of inflammatory prostaglandins, which, in turn, induced cell death. Moreover, in mice, CBD caused upregulation of inflammatory prostglandins in tumor tissue and tumor regression.

Researchers also investigated CBD-induced apoptosis in human leukemia cells. The results were similar to those detailed above, CBD made it harder for the cancerous cells to survive. CBD treatment also led to a significant decrease in tumor growth and an increase in tumor apoptosis. Consistent with the human glioma cells study, CBD exposure resulted in activation of caspases (enzymes involved in cell death), and in increase in harmful oxidants for cancerous cells.

In another study, the anti-proliferative effects of crude extract of Cannabis sativa and CBD were compared on different cervical cancer cell lines. The results were that both CBD and Cannabis sativa extracts were able to halt cell proliferation in all cell lines at varying concentrations. Further, apoptosis was induced by CBD. Overall, the data suggests that CBD, rather than crude extracts of Cannabis sativa, prevent cell growth and induce cell death in cervical cancer cell lines.

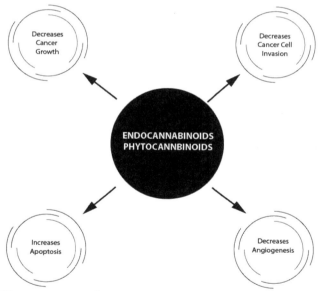

An important note: CBD may provide similar benefits with regard to multiple myeloma, a plasma cell malignancy characterized by the accumulation of a monoclonal plasma cell population in the bone marrow. The activation of a potential CBD receptor (known as TRPV2) by CBD was shown to decrease proliferation and increases susceptibility to drug-induced cell death in human cancer cells. A study published in the International Journal of Cancer found the presence of TRPV2 in multiple myeloma patients. Since the chemotherapy drug bortezomib is commonly used in multiple myeloma treatment, the effects of CBD and bortezomib in TRPV2- multiple myeloma were investigated. The results showed that CBD by itself or in synergy with bortezomib strongly inhibited growth, arrested cell cycle progression and induced multiple myeloma cell death. Furthermore, CBD exerts anti metastatic activities and has a potential to reduce carcinomas – e.g. breast, prostate tumor aggressiveness.

CANCER TREATMENT SIDE EFFECTS

One of the problems that can occur during cancer treatment, is multi-drug resistance of tumor cells (i.e. the tumor cells become resistant to the effects of the cancer drugs). As it turns out, CBD might play a crucial role in reducing multi-drug resistance in tumor cells. A recent report detailed how CBD and CBN inhibit ATP binding cassette (ABC) transporters, which contributes to the multi-drug resistance of breast tumor cells.

Chemotherapy treatment of cancer is associated with physiological side effects such as intensive vomiting. Experimental evidence from animal experiments showed that phytocannabinoids help suppress vomiting and nausea, which may be especially useful in treating symptoms of nausea and anticipatory nausea in chemotherapy patients. Research suggest that CBD acts as anti-emetic/anti-nausea effector.

Other side effects also occur with chemotherapy. For example, the chemotherapy drug paclitaxel (PAC) is associated with chemotherapy-induced neuropathic pain. In some cases, the neuropathy can lead to the discontinuation of treatment in cancer patients, even in the absence of other therapies. Since researchers previously reported that chronic administration of CBD prevents PAC-induced mechanical and thermal sensitivity in mice, they sought to determine receptor mechanisms by which CBD inhibits neuropathic pain, and whether it negatively effects nervous system function or chemotherapy efficacy. Consequently, a study was conducted with female mice to assess the ability of acute CBD pretreatment to prevent PAC-induced mechanical sensitivity (i.e. neuropathy type discomfort). The results were that administration of CBD prevented PAC-induced mechanical sensitivity.

Also, CBD + PAC combinations produce additive to synergistic inhibition of breast cancer cell viability. This data suggests that CBD is protective against PAC-induced neurotoxicity. Hence, adjunct treatment with CBD during PAC chemotherapy may be safe and effective in the prevention or treatment of chemotherapy-induced neuropathic pain. In addition, studies on the simultaneous use of CBD with radiation to treat certain cancers enhances the therapeutic effect of the treatment. Both in-vitro and in-vivo studies demonstrate the advantage of this synergistic combinational therapy to enhance the therapeutic efficacy of treatment.

ANTI-CANCER ACTION OF ENDOCANNABINOIDS AND PHYTOCANNABINOIDS (Excluding THC)

CANNABINOIDS	COMPOUND	CANCER TYPE	ANT-CANCER EFFECT	RECEPTOR INVOLVED
Endocannabinoids	Anandamide	Breast	Reduction of cancer Inhibition of cell proliferation	CB1 CB1
	Anandamide	Prostate	Inhibition of cell proliferation	CB1
Phytocannabinoids	CBD	Breast	Induction of apoptosis	CB2, TRPV1
	CBD	Prostate	Anti-proliferative and pro-apoptotic	TRPM8
	CBD	Lung	Anti-invasive action	CB2, TRPV1

With the prevalence and terminal nature of cancer, we should be open to all viable treatment options. Non-intoxicating phytocannabinoids, primarily CBD have been successfully used for various purposes in the treatment of cancers. This includes antitumor properties, drug resistance problems during cancer treatments, and diminishing cancer treatment side effects. Further ongoing research on how the ECS and phytocannabinoids regulate tumor cell growth, proliferation and death is important for the development of new therapeutic strategies for patients. The beneficial approach of providing phytocannabinoids with standard therapies may prove to be an important complementary strategy to target cancer progression while minimizing toxicity of standard treatment modalities. Nevertheless, we look forward to clinical trials to further validate efficacy in human and to finally overcome the unjustified stigma with cannabis and phytocannabinoids.

THE ENDOCANNABIDIOME & THE MICROBIOME CONNECTION FOR DIGESTIVE HEALTH

Not long ago, probiotics and the term microbiome were on the fringes of popular medicine. Fortunately, however, these are terms most of us are familiar with, thanks to widespread acceptance of the benefits of probiotics and a better understanding of the microbes lining our intestines. We have yet, as a medical community and society, to fully appreciate how the endocannabinoid system (ECS) plays a complementary role with our gut microbes in overall digestive health especially in areas to do with motility and inflammatory response. This interconnectedness between the ECS and microbiome plays into keeping a health gut/brain/immune connection that contributes immensely to our overall health.

Inside your digestive system resides approximately 1000 different species of bacteria. This collection of bacteria is known as the microbiome. These bacteria find a home primarily throughout the small and large intestines. Roughly 70% of immune activity is located in the gut, thus beneficial probiotic bacteria play an important role in immunity. Probiotic bacteria in the gut are responsible for a whole host of activities in the body including:

- Dietary fiber absorption through a fermentation process
- B-Vitamins, Vitamin K and other key nutrient creation
- Metabolic efficiency
- Healthy gut barrier maintenance

BENEFITS OF HEALTHY BACTERIA

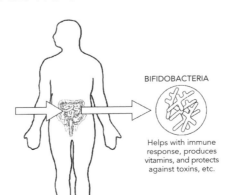

PROBIOTICS

- Protects against pathogens and toxins

- Helps absorb vitamins and minerals

- Modulates inflammatory response

BIFIDOBACTERIA

Helps with immune response, produces vitamins, and protects against toxins, etc.

LACTOBACILI

Boosts immunity, produces vitamins, and protects against toxins, etc.

OTHERS

Many other healthy family members

The gut barrier is the lining of the intestinal tract with a primary role of preventing pathogenic organisms, allergens, toxins and other harmful elements from entering the circulatory system. Should any of these destructive elements enter the body's circulatory system, it can cause a host of problematic outcomes. Gut permeability (a.k.a. "Leaky Gut Syndrome") is a disruption of this barrier protection and has been linked to many digestive diseases. Inflammatory diseases of the digestive system such as colitis are probably one of the most serious.

Researchers have been studying how supplementing probiotic bacteria can support gut barrier function. What they have found is that the beneficial bacteria protect the gut barrier by two primary methods. First, they collectively work to fight against harmful elements from potentially infiltrating the barrier. Second, the probiotic bacteria signal the cells of the gut to produce necessary protective proteins called Anti-Microbial Peptides (AMP), which work to fortify the wall. These actions together help to prevent harmful elements from entering the lining of our intestinal tract.

LEAKY GUT SYNDROME

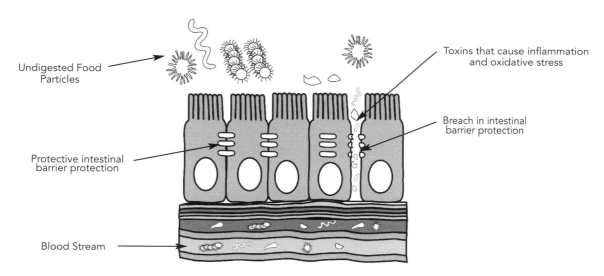

Undigested Food Particles

Toxins that cause inflammation and oxidative stress

Breach in intestinal barrier protection

Protective intestinal barrier protection

Blood Stream

Throughout life, we may take medications like antibiotics, eat the wrong foods, and anticipate life challenges. Depending on your cell makeup and the severity of the stressors on your body, the balance of beneficial probiotic bacteria in your digestive system could be disrupted. Adding probiotics to your diet, however, can help you prevent an imbalance from occurring. For this reason, probiotic supplements and foods have become very popular.

Because intestinal inflammatory conditions can be severe, it often leaves the body vulnerable to many other diseases. Over the last couple of decades, medical researchers have been trying to understand the microbiome in more depth as an effort to help treat and prevent intestinal inflammatory conditions. As a complement to the microbiome's intestinal support, new scientific research has demonstrated that the ECS plays a significant role in modulating gastrointestinal inflammation and motility. In addition, the ECS actively works to help balance the microbiome by enhancing its communication with the rest of the body.

We now understand that healthy microbes occupying our gut is vital for proper physiological functioning and overall well-being. Having more microbes in our body as compared to cells speaks to their importance in maintaining health and balance (homeostasis) in the body. In addition, our microbial environment plays a pivotal role in the tri-directional communication between the immune, nervous, and endocannabinoid systems. Several studies demonstrate how gut bacteria activates GPCR receptors that are also targeted by the ECS. In addition, specific gut microbes have been shown to have a regulatory role in increasing or decreasing ECS activity and collectively are involved in obesity, type 2 diabetes and inflammation.

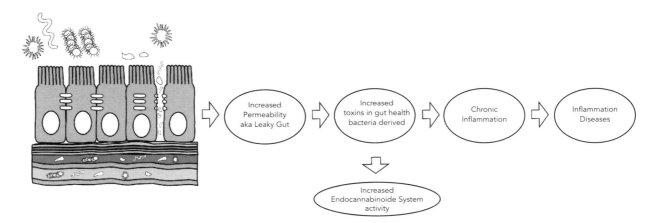

Many studies have explored the role of the microbial inhabitants of the gut in numerous conditions, especially the inflammatory disease Irritable Bowel Syndrome. When an imbalance of healthy microbes exists in our gut, it can result in a flourishing of inflammation throughout the body, increasing our risk for several degenerative conditions, and altered homeostasis. The ECS, however, plays a major role in helping regulate inflammation in key areas of the body. When tapped as a therapeutic target, the ECS assists with reducing inflammatory messengers that can wreak havoc in the body and precipitate disease.

Exploring the relationship between healthy gut bacteria and the ECS may provide clues to unlocking some of the mysteries that have eluded medical professionals for decades. The intimate interplay between probiotics, phytocannabinoids, and terpenes (organic plant compounds) work together to help fortify and maintain balance of this vital, but at times fragile, internal environment in our bodies. In addition, the use of both prebiotics (healthy fibers that feed probiotics) or probiotics in animal studies have been shown to modulate the beneficial bacterial in our gut, and, in turn, normalize ECS tone.

WELCOME TO THE ENDOCANNABIDIOME

With Germano discussing the term *Endocannabidiome*, let's help explain the workings of the ECS in the intestinal tract and revisit important aspects of this partner to the microbiome. The two primary cannabinoid receptors are called CB1 and CB2. CB1 receptors are more often responsible for stress response, relaxation, neurotransmission and involuntary motor control, while CB2 receptors are primarily focused on immunomodulatory and inflammatory response in the body. Several studies in animals and tissues of patients with a variety of gut inflammatory diseases show how the ECS gets charged up in these conditions. In particular, increased levels of the endocannabinoid anandamide (a cannabinoid produced by the body) and CB1 receptors are seen in tissue samples of those with colitis, diverticulitis, and celiac diseases. In other studies, tissue samples of patients with irritable bowel disease show enhanced expression of CB2 receptors. As with the global role of the ECS maintaining balance in the body, excitatory or excessive production of endocannabinoids are a reflection of imbalance with ensuing consequences.

GUT–BRAIN–IMMUNE–MICROBIOME–ENDOCANNABIDIOME AXIS

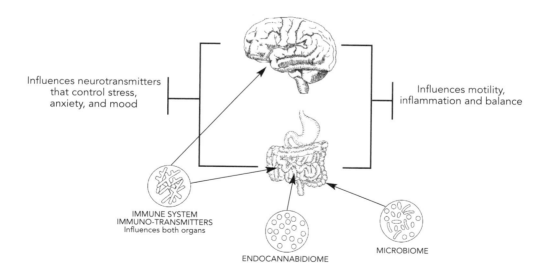

Influences neurotransmitters that control stress, anxiety, and mood

Influences motility, inflammation and balance

IMMUNE SYSTEM
IMMUNO-TRANSMITTERS
Influences both organs

ENDOCANNABIDIOME

MICROBIOME

Initially researchers found that cannabinoids such THC, which binds to the CB1 receptors, had an amazing impact on slowing motility (movements in the digestive system) especially in the presence of inflammatory related bowel diseases. When digestive inflammation is present, you will find that the motility increases and can often advance to serious bouts of diarrhea. The challenge here was that THC is an intoxicating compound that is commonly associated with the high from cannabis. For some, this is an unwanted occurrence and effect. To avoid the intoxicating presence of THC, researchers are exploring numerous other phytocannabinoids that target CB2 receptor activation that might have a similar or potentially better response without the mind altering high. A full spectrum hemp extract has been shown in many cases to provide similar benefits of THC but does not produce an inebriated state. Cannabidiol (CBD) happens to be a particular phytocannabinoid with similar non-intoxicating activity compared to THC, but beta caryophyllene (BC) specifically attaches to the CB2 receptor.

Recent research shows that CB2 receptors play a role in those specifically dealing with Inflammatory-related Bowel Diseases (IBD). Commonly associated with IBD are symptoms such as diarrhea and abdominal pain exacerbated by elevated inflammation. While research in this specific area is limited, it would follow that patients with IBD are more likely to show increased CB2 expression which is responsible to turn down the flames in the gut. More research needs to be performed but, it does indicate that activating the endocannabinoid system, more specifically CB2 expression, could help lessen pain and inflammation associated with various inflammatory bowel diseases, such as colitis.

When you consider the role of phytocannabinoids and probiotic bacteria in gut barrier protection and signaling, it only makes sense that the complementary combination of the two are key in supporting digestive health. Combining this with the fact that the CB1 and

CB1

- Decreases Acid Secretion
- Decreases Motility
- Decreases Inflammation

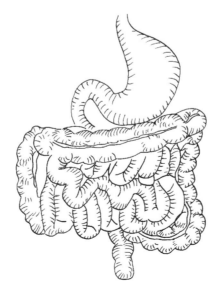

CB2

- Decreases Pain
- Decreases Inflammation
- Decreases Motility

CB2 receptor activation of the ECS helps to slow motility associated with IBD and also aids in normalizing the inflammatory process, you have the makings of an incredible strategy for treating and maintaining a healthier digestive system.

While your ECS produces its own cannabinoids called endocannabinoids but, for whatever reason, when it fails to operate correctly, plant derived cannabinoids called phytocannabinoids can be used to support the ECS. As mentioned, one of the most popular phytocannabinoids today is cannabidiol (CBD). In cell culture studies, CBD was shown to eradicate the negative effects of intestinal inflammation on permeability from inflammatory compounds. CBD affects cells in the gut called enteric glial cells (EGC). ECG's have an important role in maintaining the health and balance of the intestinal tract (homeostasis) by defending against pathogens and actively participate in the progression of intestinal inflammation.

In animal studies and tissue culture studies from patients with ulcerative colitis, CBD was shown to reduce the inflammatory/immune response and helped relax activity in gut cells by modulating the activity of ECG's involvement in inflammation. While CBD is promising in these in-vitro and in-vivo models, clinical trials will still be necessary to form a strong conclusion on their benefits. Nevertheless, we cannot ignore the entire cannabis plant by focusing only on CBD here. There are other anti-inflammatory compounds present in the plant that are in the early stages of exploration including cannabigerol (CBG) and beta caryophyllene (BC). Both have preliminary data on their potent effects on lowering inflammation via different mechanisms then CBD.

While CBD is popular and has important benefits, one should never seek just to take CBD alone or as an isolate. In fact, you want to look for products that are broader in spectrum. This means that they contain more than just CBD. Things to look for would be other cannabinoids like cannabichromene (CBC), cannabigerol (CBG), as well as beta-caryophyllene (BC). Research on BC has revealed that it has powerful immunomodulatory and gastrointestinal protective properties as well as strong anti-inflammatory and pain reduction benefits. Therefore, look for full spectrum extracts that contain CBD and other cannabinoids as well as BC.

At this moment, we have only a glimpse of how our gut bacteria controls the activity of the ECS and how our ECS is intertwined with modulating many disorders of the intestinal tract—especially the inflammatory conditions. While both our microbiome and endocannabidiome are involved in maintaining healthy permeability and barrier protection independently, it appears that collectively they work together to maintain overall gut health.

ECS & EYE HEALTH

According to the National Eye Institute, millions of people suffer from a variety of diseases affecting the eyes. Globally, close to 50% of those suffering from eye disorders are cataracts. According World Health Organization (WHO), close to 80% of global ey disorders can be prevented or controlled with early intervention and treatment. Leading the list of eye disorders are age related macular degeneration, glaucoma, and cataracts. With the prevalence of these eye diseases and others, the economic burden runs into the billions of dollars.

GLOBAL BLINDNESS

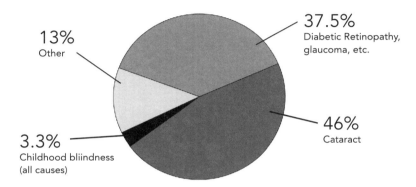

The eye is a unique organ as it is an extension of our nervous system and very much connected to our brain. In the last decade, there has been a growing interest in looking at the endocannabinoid system (ECS) and endocannabinoid functionality in the retina. In particular, researchers have been trying to understand the role the ECS plays in visual processing, function, and repair. While the ECS is a well-known physiological system focused on maintaining homeostasis and plays an important role in numerous processes, including inflammation, antioxidant and neurological protection, the potential to address the health and prevention of eye disorders is still young but very promising.

Today, we understand the numerous roles the ECS has on the health and functioning of the central nervous system (CNS). Because the eye is an extension of the CNS, it would follow that the ECS is functional in all aspects of our vision and health of ocular tissue. Researchers believe the our retinal endocannabinoid system helps to improve visual function and prevention from damage due to oxidative stress, inflammation, and excessive pressure. We've discovered that the ECS is present throughout most tissues in the eye and involved in processing visual cues reliant on our endocannabinoid receptors (CB1 and CB2) and the endocannabinoids (anandamide and 2AG). Interestingly, in humans, the levels of 2AG are significantly higher in the retina as compared to anandamide. Nevertheless, the ECS is well represented in all cell types of the eyes where they help modulate visual perception and function as well as pressure within the eye known as intraocular pressure (IOP).

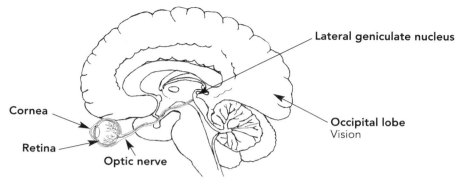

Using experimental models to explore the effects on capillaries in the retina, normal levels of both 2-AG and anandamide promote relaxing effects (vasorelaxation), whereas disrupted levels are implicated in eye disorders. There is also a growing body of evidence on the involvement of the ECS in mechanisms found in macular degeneration, glaucoma and other eye conditions. The role of the ECS in these diseases make it an important target for clinical support. Several studies also show that the number of endocannabinoids varies in eye diseases and that the ECS helps to maintain homeostasis within the entire visual system. When the eye is subject to injury, inflammation, blood pressure changes, etc., the ECS responds by fluctuating endocannabinoids to help restore balance in the eye and to prevent premature retinal cells from dying (apoptosis). For overall ocular health and protection, it is important to tap into the ECS for strategies to restore normal levels of endocannabinoids in the eye, modify ECS regulation of IOP, and increase the survival of retinal cells. Nevertheless, we are still in the early stages of understanding the relationship of ECS fluctuations in various eye disorders and look forward to eventual clinical trials.

Glaucoma, a neurodegenerative disease defined by elevation of IPO and loss of retinal cells, is a major cause of blindness. While THC (a CB1 agonist) has been shown to reduce IOP in a few human studies, its intoxicating effects prevent it from being a primary phytocannabinoid strategy in some patients. However, non-intoxicating compounds that attach to the CB receptors were found in pre-clinical studies to be successful in reducing IOP and inflammation as well. There is other interesting work to show that aside from modulating the IOP in the eye, the ECS, through its neuroprotective effects, helps reduce retinal cell damage and loss. This is particularly important for glaucoma.

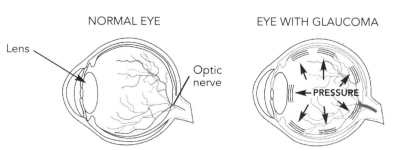

Because the ECS plays critical roles in controlling oxidative stress and inflammation, its effects are especially important for treating eye diseases. Several inflammatory components (cytokines, tumor necrosis factor, etc.) and elevated oxidants contribute heavily to the degree of glaucoma and uveitis (inflammation of the middle eye), but with alterations of the ECS, patients can see relief from these conditions. Age related macular degeneration and diabetic retinopathy (DR) can also be relieved by targeting the ECS, this is because elevated inflammatory markers and neurodegeneration are part of the etiology (the processes that cause the disorder), and the ECS plays a vital role in regulating inflammation and neurodegeneration. In animals with DR, studies revealed that chronic administration of cannabidiol (CBD) reduced all inflammatory and oxidative stress issues responsible for retinal cell death. CBD was instrumental in resolving the deleterious issues seen in DR by influencing receptor activity that is implicated in various eye diseases. On the other hand, activating the CB2 receptor specifically plays into the anti-inflammatory attributes of the ECS including its ocular effects.

The cells in the eye that respond to light are called photoreceptors. These cells are also a major target for disruption in many retinal diseases. In studies where animals were exposed to bright light, the use of various antioxidants and phytochemicals were capable of reducing the destruction of photoreceptors. Very bright light can stimulate photoreceptors in the eye to prematurely die. The herb saffron, surprisingly, is capable of reducing this effect. In humans, saffron was shown to be very effective in reducing retinal damage and preserve functionality in ocular tissue as well. Saffron's mechanism of action points to its effects on influencing certain genes associated with controlling the progression of eye damage by activating antioxidant and anti-inflammatory neuroprotective effects. While CB2 receptors are involved in protecting eyes from very bright light exposure, animal studies show that elevated overexpression of CB receptors are implicated in ocular diseases. Saffron helps to down-regulate excitatory CB1 and CB2 activity when exposed to very bright light which has potential in treating diseases of the retina.

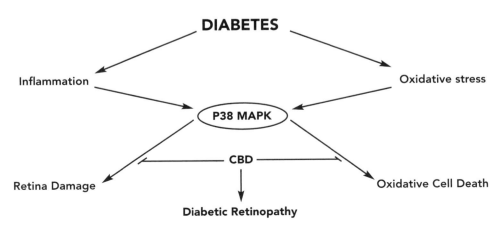

In addition to saffron, CBD was also shown, in several animal studies, to protect the retina from destructive excitatory behavior and provided protection from increased inflammatory components in the eye. It is well understood that diabetes causes significant oxidative stress and accumulation of toxic glutamate in the eye. CBD was also shown to increase enzymes that break down glutamate and preserving retinal functioning in diabetic animals. Studies also demonstrate that CBD blocks an enzyme called p38MAPK that damages the retina and increases cell death in diabetes. The p38MAPK enzyme is involved in controlling several cellular responses to inflammation and stress. Elevations of this enzyme are implicated in several effects that can damage tissues and CBD quiets its activity. Additionally, CBD prevents neurodegeneration via antioxidant and anti-inflammatory expression and protected retinal cells in animal models of diabetic retinopathy. While lutein, zeaxanthin, quercetin, many of the compounds in the polyphenol family, and vitamins are important for eye function, it is just as important to include full spectrum CBD oil as a primary player to support the endocannabinoid systems role in ocular health.

ECS &
NEUROLOGICAL HEALTH

The brain is the body's most complex organ and, despite its compact three-pound size, it commands everything from memory to sex drive. Maintaining the health of your brain is important for an array of reasons; not least of which, as we age, all of us lose brain cells as a result of genetic weaknesses, infections, drugs, poor diet, injury, and environmental toxins. The combination of these effects on the brain are often a contributor to neurological disease and dysfunction, especially in later years of our life. Millions of people suffer from the ravages of brain/mental illnesses each year. So, it is little wonder that many of us have accepted the notion that we are fated to suffer neurological diseases and lose brain function as we age. Well, maybe not!

New investigations into the role of the endocannabinoid system (ECS) in our brain and its relationship in numerous neurological diseases is leading us down a different perspective – keeping a healthy functioning ECS is the key to keeping your brain healthy! We have only begun to understand the intricate dance between the ECS, the brain, and their modulating effects that influence the entire body and how targeting the ECS is useful in the treatment of many neurological illnesses. The ECS is one of the most extensive signaling systems in our brain and it assists in the regulation of numerous neurological effects, such as:

- Providing neurons (brain cells) to be more adaptogenic and provides greater flexibility for them to adjust to injury, disease or environmental changes.
- Protecting the brain from toxic excitatory expression of glutamate. Excessive glutamate release in the brain can lead to death of neurons.
- Protecting the brain from the deleterious effects of inflammatory components as a result from oxidative stress, inflammatory cytokines from the immune system, etc.
- Modulating neurotransmitter release, reduces oxidative stress, involved in pain signaling.

NEUROLOGICAL DISEASES

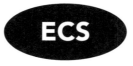

PHYSIOLOGICAL FUNCTIONS

- Epilepsy
- Alzheimers/Dimentia
- Multiple Sclerosis
- Parkinsons
- Tramatic brain injury

- Builds brain cells
- Improves memory
- Reduces inflammation
- Reduces oxidative stress
- Governs neurotransmission

Dr. Mechoulam's research into the interaction of tetrahydrocannabinol (THC) in the brain was a milestone in cannabinoid research and happens to be the impetus behind the evolving field of cannabinoid medicine and the discovery of the ECS. While THC has numerous medicinal benefits, the intoxicating effects and legality issues hamper its use. While Dr. Mechoulam graced us with important discoveries in the 1960s on the isolation and detection of THC and how it interacts with CB1 receptors, we have since come to understand the inner workings of the ECS with respect to both endocannabinoids and phytocannabinoids (such as cannabidiol, etc.).

When it comes to our cannabinoid receptors, both CB1 and CB2 receptors coexist in the central nervous system (CNS) and perform and modulate all of our neurological events. For example, CB receptors are concentrated in key functional areas such as the basal ganglia (movement), cerebral cortex (cognition), cerebellum (movement), hippocampus (memory, stress), spinal cord (pain signaling), and others. Since CB2 receptor activation results in anti-inflammatory activity and does not cause intoxicating effects, it has become a target for further study into the treatment of certain neurological diseases including Alzheimer's (AD) and multiple sclerosis (MS).

CONCENTRATIONS OF CB RECEPTORS

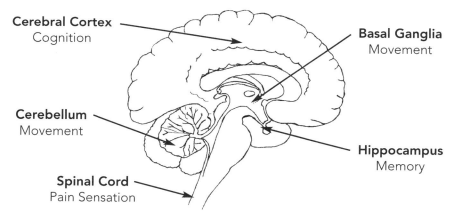

In AD patients, researchers have discovered plaques, or patches of dead cells and other castoff material, lying outside the brains neurons. Most of these plaques are located in areas of the brain associated with memory. At the core of these plaques is a potentially deadly substance called beta amyloid, an abnormal protein not usually found in the brain. Adding insult to injury, an overzealous immune system contributes to increased inflammatory messengers that contribute to oxidative stress and beta amyloid. The result is a complete disruption of the intricate process of communication between neurons (brain cells). The disruption is caused either by poor neuron function or cell death as a result of several pathological factors noted above. In preclinical AD studies, CB2 receptor activation is involved in providing treatment support by reducing invasive neuroinflammation and increasing the removal of harmful amyloid plaque deposits - both of which contribute to the ultimate demise of brain cells. In other in vitro and in vivo studies, therapeutic uses of cannabidiol (CBD) or a combination of CBD and THC showed demonstrable improvements.

Although MS is categorized as a neurological disease, it is also a disease of the immune system. In patients with MS, the immune system turns against the body instead of defending it which technically can be classified as an autoimmune disease. The very term multiple sclerosis literally means "many scars" and refers to the scarring (or plaques) on nerve fibers in the brain and spinal cord. The inflammation in the nerve fibers wears away the protective myelin insulation causing a disruption in the high speed transmission of electrical messages between the CNS and the rest of the body. In preclinical MS studies, the therapeutic target of activating effect of CB2 receptors resulted in modulating the inflammatory component of the disease. In addition, enhanced CB2 activity helped serve as a marker for identifying MS plaques that can be helpful in pinpoint targeting therapy.

In AD and MS tissue culture and animal studies, CB2 receptors have been shown to be part of the neuroprotective activity of the ECS. Findings from human brain tissue suggests that increased CB2 receptor activity is a common response to inflammatory triggered brain injury seen in these diseases. Also, variation of 2AG or anandamide levels in the CNS are important findings as they alter brain functionality and protection. These observations have not only been seen in AD and MS, but also in the blood of patients with Amyotrophic lateral sclerosis (ALS), Huntington's, and Parkinson's diseases.

In Parkinson's disease (PD), the typical tremors, slowness of movement, and rigidity is clearly linked to a progressive deterioration of dopamine producing cells and neuroinflammation in the brain. Dopamine is a neurotransmitter that controls movement and balance in the body, among other important functions. Scientists also believe there is a genetic impairment in the ability for brain cells to rid themselves of toxins are the key reason why certain people are at risk for PD. When neurons are unable to naturally neutralize toxins, the immune system begins to mount its forces against those invaders which may result in further destruction of brain cells from inflammation and oxidative stress. In preclinical studies, 2Ag levels were significantly increased when the known neurotoxin MPP (1-methyl-4-phenyl-1,2,3,6-tetrahydropyridine) was administered to animals. 2AG is known to reduce expression of inflammation and is concentrated in areas of the brain affected by PD. The 2AG treated animals displayed neuroprotective effects including reduced loss of dopamine levels, inhibited expression of inflammatory and oxidative markers.

Globally, over the past few decades, neurological disorders have significantly increased and rank as one of the leading causes of death and disability. Several studies over the past decade help support the role the ECS plays in the etiology (the cause) of many neurological diseases. When the ECS is over or underactive, the brain and CNS feels its effects — positively or negatively, depending on the nature of the activity. An imbalance of ECS activity is a common and prevalent neurological effect seen in dementia conditions, stroke, Parkinson's, multiple sclerosis, brain trauma, and epilepsy.

In studies of patients with epilepsy, researchers found reduced levels of anandamide and lower numbers of CB1 receptors. Given that anandamide and CB1 receptors have been found to contribute to anti-seizure activity, it seems then that finding ways to normalize healthy levels of both would help treat epilepsy symptoms. Interestingly, the use of cannabis preparations to treat epilepsy dates back to the 1800's where Indian hemp provided noteworthy success. Fast forward to the present, CBD preparations have being used in several human trails with notable success. CBD is able to raise anandamide levels, which can reduce inflammation, oxidative stress, and excitability in the brain. Further, CBD helps provide cellular calcium ion balance which is another important mechanism to treating seizure activity. GW Pharmaceuticals FDA approved CBD drug called Epidiolex has shown promise in reducing the number of seizures in patients with epilepsy. More studies are ongoing, so we are likely to learn more in the near future. Additionally, GW's Sativex drug (combination THC and CBD) has been used successfully in clinical trials in patients with MS to alleviate neuropathic pain and spasticity/spasms.

CANNABIDIOL IN THE CNS

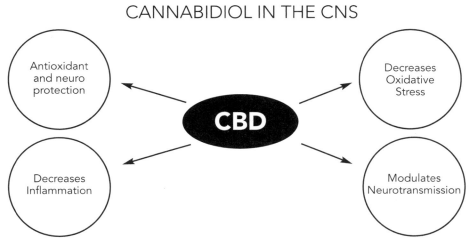

In 2013, the US government Department of Health & Human Services was issued a patent titled "Cannabinoids as Antioxidants and Neuroprotectants". This patent outlined the neuroprotective effects of non-intoxicating cannabinoids, such as CBD, that can limit further neurological damage following stroke or trauma or in the treatment of several neurodegenerative diseases. Traumatic brain injury, as a result of unfortunate accidents, is very prevalent yet lacks efficient therapeutic strategies. At the cellular level, we see the same milieu as seen in neurodegenerative diseases – inflammation, neuronal death, oxidative stress, glutamate toxicity, and others.

Preclinical animal studies show how the ECS plays a major role in protecting the brain from the deleterious effects of inflammation. Increased amounts of inflammation is not only destructive itself, but also increases the permeability of our cells, which can cause premature cell death. Researchers also studied the role of 2AG in lowering inflammation and the toxic effects of excess glutamate activity in the brain. When animals were treated with compounds known to block the enzyme that degrades 2AG, they saw a reduction in neurotoxic excitability and normalization of glutamate involvement. In short, they demonstrated that the ECS provides neuroprotection on several levels. The effect of 2AG also demonstrates its participation in supporting homeostasis in brain cells and helps them adapt to the insult of injury.

Further investigation takes us a bit deeper in our understanding of the role of endocannabinoids in the body. Other than direct activity of anandamide or 2AG, inhibiting further damage to brain from inflammation and oxidative stress were shown to be a result of endocannabinoids producing other important modulators of inflammation including prostaglandins (a group of fats that play major roles in either increasing or decreasing inflammation). Additionally, anandamide and 2AG affect other receptors besides CB1 and CB2 including TRPV1, GABA or PPAR receptors that are involved in neurological health by also modulating inflammation and glutamate toxicity.

Maintaining homeostasis in the brain and CNS is paramount to its health and disturbances in its balance is commonly seen in all neurodegenerative diseases. Of all the systems in the body to assist in healthy functioning and repair, the ECS is the most important due to its modulating effects on producing new brain cells to neuroprotection (anti-inflammatory, antioxidant). Strengthening and supporting normal functioning of the ECS helps to alleviate the pathology in the brain as seen in many models of brain disorders including Alzheimer's, multiple sclerosis, Parkinson's, epilepsy, and brain injury. The operative word here is "normal functioning" as either insufficient or excessive activation of the ECS is not warranted. While numerous preclinical studies have enriched our understanding of the role the ECS plays in brain diseases, we look towards continued clinical trials to broaden our insights for clinical application. Unfortunately, several of the clinical trials utilized drugs consisting of single magic bullet cannabinoids. As previously noted in this book, other phytocannabinoids in hemp are equal if not more important than just CBD or THC including cannabigerol (CBG), beta caryophyllene, and others. In a few studies and in clinical practice, when a full entourage of phytocannabinoids were compared to CBD isolate alone in patients, clinical outcome with the group utilizing more than just CBD isolate was significantly better. It would therefore make sense to investigate full spectrum phytocannabinoid preparations in clinical trials addressing neurodegenerative diseases.

CBD, HEMP & ITS FAMILY OF PHYTOCANNABINOIDS

While the terms marijuana and industrial hemp have been mistakenly used to describe each other for decades, it is important to distinguish the differences between both of these important plants. From a botanical standpoint, they are classified as Cannabis sativa, but that is where the similarity ends. Both plants are visually distinct and different with marijuana being shorter, squattier, and broader leaves while hemp is very tall, long stalks, and narrower leaves. In addition, marijuana is commonly cultivated for its intoxicating phytocannabinoid THC (tetrahydrocannabinol) for its recreational and medicinal applications. Yes, medical applications! As history will show, aside from its use in traditional medicine, several pharmaceutical preparations have been commercialized in the past that utilized THC for its analgesic effects. Nevertheless, THC and marijuana have legal constraints.

MARIJUANA vs INDUSTRIAL HEMP PLANT VISUAL DISTINCTION

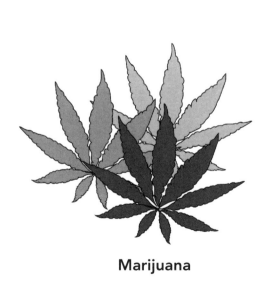

Marijuana

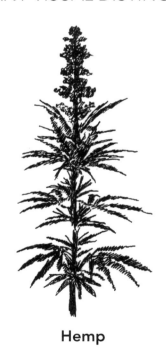

Hemp

On the other hand, industrial hemp has been cultivated as an important agricultural crop throughout history for its use as food, clothing, fiber, fuel, building materials and medicines as well. Let us not forget that our forefathers grew industrial hemp and depended on it for many purposes (clothing, fiber, food, etc.), our Declaration of Independence was written on paper made from it, Henry Ford built the first car whose structure and fuel utilized hemp, and during World War II a major "Hemp for Victory" media campaign was instituted encouraging farmers to grow this important plant. Today, technological advances utilizing industrial hemp have expanded its use to include the production of plastics, concrete (hempcrete), printer filaments, and more. Also, ultra-strong hemp nano sheets were used to manufacture entire shells of vehicles and featured on Jay Leno's Garage TV program.

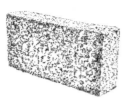

HEMPcrete

- Environmentally friendly
- Better sound proofing
- Cost effective
- Insect/rat resistant
- Fireproof and earthquake resistant
- Low maintenance

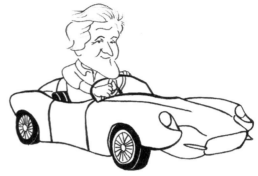

HEMP is Stronger Than Steel

- Environmentally friendly
- Lighter
- More efficient

While all of these attributes places hemp as one of the most import agricultural plants on our planet, its unjustified ban in the Marijuana Tax Act of 1937 and absurd placement in the Controlled Substances Act has kept us in the dark ages. Fortunately, in December 2018, the Farm Bill (Agriculture Improvement Act of 2018) was signed into law and the groundless handcuffs on hemp were finally lifted. In addition to hemp's significant agricultural contributions, there are over 100 botanical compounds found in its leaves, flower, and stalk known as phytocannabinoids – the non-intoxicating type that don't get you high, but have tremendous medicinal value in the body.

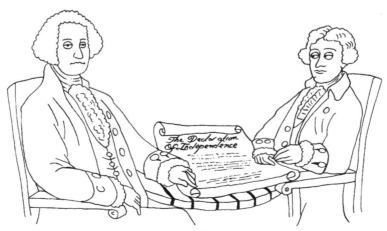

The phytocannabinoid class of naturally occurring compounds found in hemp interact in a variety of ways with our body's endocannabinoid system. Some are direct agonists to our receptors while others act indirectly. For example, CBD does not attach to the CB1 and CB2 receptors, but indirectly supports CB1 receptors by inhibiting the breakdown of anandamide which attaches to CB1. On the other hand, beta caryophyllene, a minor phytocannabinoid in hemp, is a strong agonist to the CB2 receptor. Therefore, if one truly wants to benefit by supporting the whole ECS, taking CBD alone will not do so. Unfortunately, we have been focusing only on CBD (cannabidiol) which represents just one of over 100 important phytocannabinoids. While CBD is the most dominant phytocannabinoid in hemp, the others are important – some more important than CBD!

Collectively, the entire class of phytocannabinoids synergistically gives rise to hemp's clinical importance in the body. The collective of compounds in cannabis that work together as a family to produce more effective benefits as compared to isolating one was discussed by Dr. Mechoulam in the 1980's. He addresses the single magic bullet issue by stating that the synergism in the plants full complement of active compounds plays a role in the widely held view that plants are better agents than the natural products isolated from them!

Further establishing the synergistic benefits of the whole plant was beautifully elucidated in a published paper in the British Journal of Pharmacology by Dr. Ethan Russo titled "Taming THC: potential cannabis synergy and phytocannabinoid-terpenoid entourage effects." He discussed how all of the phytocannabinoids and terpenes in cannabis have unique properties that contribute to the plant's clinical benefits and their synergistic effects are greater than any single magic bullet approach.

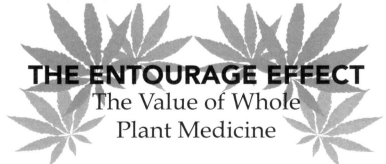

THE ENTOURAGE EFFECT
The Value of Whole
Plant Medicine

"The whole is greater than the sum of its parts." - Aristotle

From a botanical medicine point of view, dietary herbal supplements have always followed this philosophy and most herbal plants contain numerous active synergistic components. Yes, CBD is incredibly important, having tremendous medical value. Nevertheless, it is important to recognize and appreciate the entire family and what the whole plant offers as a full spectrum extract.

MEET THE FAMILY

Besides the agricultural benefits of Cannabis sativa, the plant has a cornucopia of active compounds including phytocannabinoids and terpenes. In marijuana, the most dominant phytocannabinoid is THC (tetrahydrocannabinol) an intoxicating compound that has both recreational and medical value. In hemp, the dominant phytocannabinoid is CBD (cannabidiol) that has numerous beneficial effects including anticonvulsant, anti-inflammatory, muscle relaxant, antianxiety, and neuroprotective. While it is the most dominant and has medicinal value, it is not alone. The remaining 90+ phytocannabinoids may be minor in number in the plant, but collectively has major clinical value. Before I focus on CBD, here are some quick notes about a few members of the family of phytocannabinoids:

- **Beta Caryophyllene (BCP)** – a potent CB2 agonist which makes it a perfect complement to CBD. Attaching to the CB2 receptor provides for significant anti-in flammatory effects both orally and topically.

- **Cannabigerol (CBG)** – the precursor to CBD, CBC, and THC. In preclinical studies, CBG has been shown to act as a neuroprotectant, has anti-bacterial activity, reduces intraocular pressure in the eyes, inhibits cancer cell growth, promotes bone growth, acts as a muscle relaxant, and helps decrease inflammation.

- **Cannabichromene (CBC)** – works with both endocannabinoid and non cannabinoid receptors in the body including the TRPV's. In preclinical studies, CBC has been shown to relieve pain, anti-depressant effects, has anti-inflammatory and antioxidant activity, promotes bone growth, acts as a neuroprotectant, and has potent anti-cancer effects.

- **Cannabinol (CBN)** – produced from the breakdown of THC. Preclinical studies show it has mild intoxicating sedative effects, anti-epileptic effects, promotes bone growth, aids in sleep by prolonging sleep time, may reduce pain and muscle spasms, anti-inflammatory and acts as an antibacterial and lowers intraocular pressure when applied topically.

- **Cannabidivarin (CBDV)** – works with both endocannabinoid and non cannabinoid receptors in the body including TRPV1. In preclinical studies, CBDV has been shown to reduce excitability in the brain, modulate gene expression and has promise in the treatment of epilepsy.

… and then there is **Cannabidiol (CBD)**:

CBD is the most dominant phytocannabinoid in hemp and has a significant history in scientific circles as it has been the most studied outside of THC. Its clinical benefits requires an entire book to completely review and outside the realms of this beginners guide. There is a wealth of scholarly work published in the scientific community to review and enjoy. Much of the initial human research has been on its use as an anti-convulsant, anti-epileptic agent using GW Pharmaceuticals Epidiolox® (CBD only) and for treating cancer symptoms with Sativex® (THC, CBD). CBD has been shown to effectively suppress seizure activity and used successfully in children and adults. Doses of CBD in the several hundred milligram range was used in children with Dravet Syndrome as well as those with treatment resistant forms of the disease as well. Today, CBD research is going on at a feverish pace due to its abundant biochemical and physiological effects and clinical importance.

As a summary, CBD does not securely attach to the endocannabinoid receptors (CB1, CB2). It does prevent certain molecules from attaching to the CB1 receptor such as THC but performs many other functions in the body. One very meaningful functions of CBD is to maintain endocannabinoid tone. It does this by interfering with the FAAH enzyme that degrades anandamide. In the beginning chapters of this book, you learned how important anandamide is in the body!

In preclinical studies, CBD has been shown to elicit anti-inflammatory effects in a variety of ways including decreasing production of certain inflammatory compounds such as tumor necrosis factor alpha (major inflammatory component in arthritis) and other cytokines (cells secreted by the immune system that can cause inflammation). In terms of pain relief, CBD can also attach to the opioid receptors in the body and may play a part in overall activity of opioid activation. So as a pain reliever, CBD can quell both nerve pain (pain sensation) and pain associated with inflammation. Just as our endocannabinoids anandamide and 2AG are promiscuous by influencing other non-cannabinoid receptors in the body, CBD does the same. CBD has an affinity to 5HT1a receptors where it helps in increasing blood flow to the brain. In addition, by increasing superoxide dismutase (SOD), its potent antioxidant capabilities suggests its usefulness as a neuroprotectant with potential use in neurodegenerative diseases. While there are many preclinical studies demonstrating CBD's neurological benefits, findings on how CBD increased cell survival after exposure to beta amyloid (destructive protein seen in Alzheimer's disease) shows promise as an adjunct treatment.

There are several preclinical and clinical trials demonstrating CBD's anti-anxiety effects in healthy normal subjects as well as those with clinical social anxiety. CBD exerts anxiolytic effects in several areas of the brain in a variety of doses. Typical doses of from 300mgs – 600mgs CBD were reported to have significant beneficial effects in humans without any adverse reactions. At lower doses, 25mgs CBD resulted in improvements of all symptoms of anxiety with a side benefit of reported better sleep in humans. The effects of CBD on sleep are very interesting in that the dose follows a bi-phasic response. Small amounts of CBD (15mgs) have more of an uplifting effect, while larger doses (150mgs+) increases total sleep time. Additional studies had mixed results in that high doses did not have an effect. Animal models of Post Traumatic Stress Disorder (PTSD) have shown that CBD can both facilitate the extinction of aversive memories and block their reconsolidation. As seen in animals, recent human studies have confirmed the ability of 25 – 32mgs of CBD to alter aversive memories and blocked their recall and provided major improvements in the PTSD symptoms.

Finally, the potential of CBD as an anti-cancer agent has been studied in several cancer cell lines with very promising results as discussed in a previous chapter. CBD consistently shows its cancer fighting properties via increasing apoptosis (cell death) in cancer cells and by strangling the tumor by inhibiting its blood supply and may potentially be an effective adjunct to traditional treatment.

Human and animals studies have offered compelling data to show that CBD offers therapeutic benefits for many disorders. The effects of CBD in the body are many and work at different stages and receptor sites. CBD also has several mechanisms of action that account for its diverse beneficial effects with the advantage of having good tolerance and few adverse reactions. However, even in the face of positive evidence CBD has on the ECS and potential in health and disease, more clinical studies are necessary to grasp a better understanding of its efficacy.

To be continued …

FULL SPECTRUM HEMP vs. CBD ISOLATE

While hemp (cannabis sativa (C. sativa)) has been used in traditional medicine since ancient times, modern medicine has only recently appreciated its healing qualities. The discovery of the endocannabinoid system (ECS) in mammals at the end of the twentieth century, as well as the finding of exogenous phytocannabinoids in hemp (cannabis), allowed the scientific community to better understand the clinical relevancy of this important class of compounds. Over the last few decades, the literature indicates that phytocannabinoids are valuable medicinal products in the therapy of numerous pathophysiological conditions, such as inflammatory diseases, neurodegenerative diseases, gastrointestinal, metabolic and cardiovascular diseases, and cancer. Moreover, cannabis sativa has pain relieving qualities, as discussed in other chapters of this book.

In using standard marijuana extracts, the extraction process typically leaves undesirable intoxicating psychotropic effects. These psychotropic consequences appear after administration of specific phytocannabinoid compounds, such as tetrahydrocannabinol (THC). An important way to avoid these undesirable outcomes is to utilize hemp-derived phytocannabinoid extracts containing little to no intoxicating THC. Recently, extracts of hemp derived phytocannabinoids with little to no trace of psychoactive THC have enthusiastically entered the marketplace. One important phytocannabinoid with potential therapeutic significance but lacking intoxicating activity is cannabidiol (CBD). Many recent studies have primarily utilized CBD as an isolate of the plant (80 – 99% pure CBD), fewer have explored a full spectrum botanical concentrate - especially varieties rich in CBD. While CBD has antipsychotic, neuroprotective, anti-inflammatory, anti-anxiety, and antioxidant activity, reduces somatic symptoms accompanying anxiety states, etc., it seems that its antiepileptic effect has been mostly studied and reported in the literature. Because of its enormous importance in the human body, the question arises whether the attainment of therapeutic effects are best provided by the administration of a purified CBD isolate or as part of a full spectrum of phytocannabinoids as naturally found in the plant.

In well-established traditional herbal medical therapies, including Traditional Chinese and Ayurveda Medicine, full spectrum herbal extracts have long been favored in place of single components isolated from plants. Full spectrum allows for synergistic interactions or multi-factorial effects between a variety of components present in plants. The practice of isolating compounds from plants began as a Western medical practice and is the foundation for modern Western medicines. While isolates are preferred for their high activity, they have disadvantages. First, it is important to understand that in any disease or condition, there are many pathways contributing to the etiology, or cause, of the illness. Unfortunately, there is no one single drug, nutrient or plant compound that can address all the pathways to a disease. Current Wholistic Medicine has embraced the multiple pathway approach to disease and appreciates the synergism of the full spectrum of a plant's makeup. Unfortunately, Western medicine practice has struggled to find ways to utilize the full complement of ingredients naturally occurring in plants.

Further, isolates from plants rarely have the same degree of activity as the whole plant complex at comparable concentrations or dosages of the single active component. This phenomenon in isolates is attributed to the absence of interacting substances present in the full spectrum extract. When we look at the effects of plant constituents in the body, many have been shown to act at on either different receptors, pathways, and or targets - making their therapeutic effects multi-faceted when being administered to treat a given disease or condition. The collective of actives in the plant may also improve bioavailability or enhance a desired effect that cannot be achieved by singling out one ingredient.

Numerous observations accumulated over millennia on the therapeutic use of herbal medicines demonstrate that natural complexes of botanical substances found in plants are often characterized by enhanced efficacy as compared to individual active ingredients isolated from them. This has been exemplified in the medicinal practices of ancient China, India or Mesopotamia, and seems to have a place in relation to the ingredients found in cannabis. This is true for all other herbal supplements, we do not try to isolate specific compounds. Why? There is not one ginsenoside in ginseng; there is not one isobutylamide in Echinacea; there is not one ginkgolide in ginkgo; there is not one curcuminoid in curcumin. So, why are we fixated on the myopic thinking that there is one phytocannabinoid (CBD) in hemp?

The truth is there are over 100 phytocannabinoids in hemp, and CBD is not responsible for all of the plant's beneficial activity. Dr. Mechoulam said it best when he stated that: "Biochemically active natural products, are in many instances accompanied by chemically related though biologically inactive constituents. Very seldom is the biological activity of the active constituent assayed together with inactive 'entourage' compounds. Investigations of the effect of the active component in the presence of its 'entourage' compounds may lead to results that differ from those observed with the active component only."

As mentioned before, taking plants and trying to isolate the compounds may seem like an effective way to treat, but limitations are significant. Understanding the complexity and synergism in plants rather than trying to isolate pure single compounds, however, goes against the reductionist philosophy of western medical thought. It's time for us to move beyond this myopic thinking. The intimate synergy between the action of several plant components is known to achieve an effect greater than any single component. The simultaneous interaction of numerous valuable phyto-cannabinoids contained in hemp/cannabis extracts seems to mutually intensify/modulate their activity.

In addition to the large family of 100+ phytocannabinoids found in cannabis (CBD, CBG, CBC, CBN, etc.), there also exists the family of terpenes (close to 200) – the active components that give the smell and taste of many plants. Both terpenes and phytocannabinoids are produced inside cannabis with the most common and studied beta caryophyllene (a CB2 agonist), limonene, myrcene, humulene, alpha-pinene, and linalool. It is believed that the combination of both classes of compounds work together and are responsible for the anti-inflammatory/pain, anti-anxiety, anti-cancer, etc. effects of the plant. With reference to phytocannabinoids in the literature, studies gradually appear to prove the therapeutic advantage of whole plant full spectrum extracts over purified single cannabinoid compounds, including CBD.

Research on mice that were administered standardized full spectrum cannabis extracts (intraperitoneally or orally) dose-dependently saw anti-inflammatory and analgesic (pain relief) activities. In contrast, after administration of purified CBD a bell–shaped dose–response was observed, which limited its therapeutic effects. Moreover, the full spectrum extract reduced not only pain, but also significantly prevented pro-inflammatory cytokine TNFα production in vivo. It is interesting to note that at least 25 mg/kg full spectrum extract, which corresponds to about 5 mg CBD, was required to achieve the anti-inflammatory effect. Authors suggested that other components in the full spectrum extract synergize with CBD to achieve the anti-inflammatory action greater than when using CBD isolate alone. In addition, it may have contributed to overcoming the bell-shaped dose-response of purified CBD. Authors concluded that full spectrum extract is superior over CBD for the treatment of inflammatory conditions.

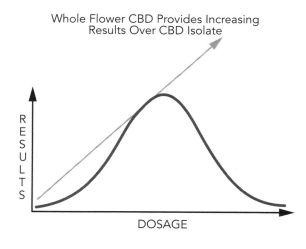

Whole Flower CBD Provides Increasing Results Over CBD Isolate

RESULTS

DOSAGE

In other in vitro studies, standardized cannabis full spectrum extracts produced a stronger inhibitory effect on animal and human bladder contractility in comparison to pure CBD isolate. In preclinical treatment of multiple sclerosis (MS) there was a clear advantage of full spectrum extract efficacy over pure CBD isolate to treat urinary urgency, incontinence episodes, frequency, and nocturia. A 2018 meta-analysis published study (11 valid references, data of a total of 670 patients) compared the potential

There Is MoreThere Is More Than Just One Ginsenoside In Ginseng

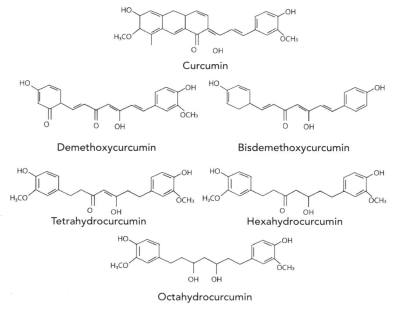

Ginsenoside Rb1

Ginsenoside Rg1

Ginsenoside Re

Ginsenoside Rh2

Ginsenoside Rd

Ginsenoside Rh1

Compound K

Compound Rg2

Ginsenoside Rg3

Ginsenoside Rf

Ginsenoside F1

Ginsenoside Ro

There Is More Than One Curcuminoid In Curcumin

Curcumin

Demethoxycurcumin

Bisdemethoxycurcumin

Tetrahydrocurcumin

Hexahydrocurcumin

Octahydrocurcumin

There Is More Than One Ginkgolide In Ginkgo

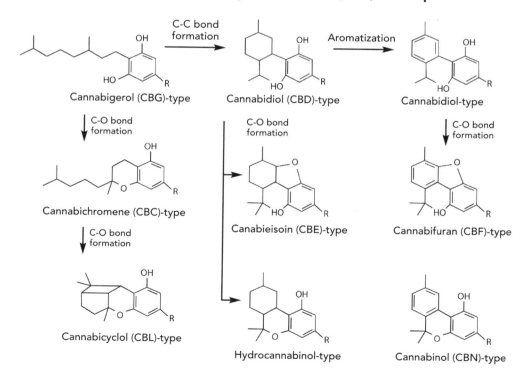

Ginkgolide A
Ginkgolide B
Ginkgolide C
Ginkgolide J
Ginkgolide M

Ginkgolide K
Ginkgolide L

Bilobalide (BL)

So Why Would One Think There Is Only One Phytocannabinoid (CBD) In Hemp?

Cannabigerol (CBG)-type

C-C bond formation →

Cannabidiol (CBD)-type

Aromatization →

Cannabidiol-type

C-O bond formation ↓

Cannabichromene (CBC)-type

C-O bond formation

Canabieisoin (CBE)-type

C-O bond formation ↓

Cannabifuran (CBF)-type

C-O bond formation ↓

Cannabicyclol (CBL)-type

Hydrocannabinol-type

Cannabinol (CBN)-type

therapeutic properties of CBD alone with CBD-rich full spectrum cannabis extracts in treating refractory (treatment-resistant) epilepsy in humans. It is worth noting that the daily average dose in patients using full-plant extracts was more than four times lower than of those using purified CBD. Almost two thirds of patients reported improvement in the frequency of seizures. Moreover, the reports of mild and severe adverse effects were more frequent in products containing purified CBD than in CBD-rich full spectrum extracts. Authors concluded that full spectrum CBD-rich extracts seem to present a better therapeutic profile than purified CBD isolate and the roots of this difference is likely due to synergistic effects of CBD with other related phytocannabinoid and terpene compounds. In fact, in the literature there are very few studies in which the authors failed to show differences in the use of preparations from whole plants relative to purified single cannabinoids.

In summary, the data proposed by researchers shows that the use of full spectrum cannabis extracts containing the entire group of active ingredients found naturally occurring in cannabis with simultaneous reduction in the content of intoxicating ingredients seems justified. Moreover, a growing number of studies also points to the advantage of the full spectrum extracts over isolated phytocannabinoids administered individually. However, further support of the superiority of whole plant cannabis products over single compounds requires more research, especially for specific therapeutic applications.

APPENDIX

YOUR AMAZING BODY

The Embodied Mind: A review on functional genomic and neurological correlates of mind-body therapies., Muehsam D, Lutgendorf S, Mills PJ, Rickhi B, Chevalier G, Bat N, Chopra D, Gurfein B., Neurosci Biobehav Rev. 2017 Feb; 73:165-181.

Psychoneuroimmunology: The Experiential Dimension., Ulvestad E., Methods Mol Biol. 2012; 934:21-37.

Clinical Psychoneuroimmunology., Irwin MR, Rothermundt M., Handb Clin Neurol. 2012; 106:211-25.

Epigenetics and Psychoneuroimmunology: Mechanisms and Models., Mathews HL, Janusek LW., Brain Behav Immun. 2011 Jan; 25 (1):25-39.

The Mind-body Connection: Not Just a Theory Anymore., Littrell J., Soc Work Health Care. 2008; 46(4):17-37.

Jay Lombard, DO: *Exploring the Brain-Mind-Body Connection.* Interview by Frank Lampe and Suzanne Snyder., Lombard J., Altern Ther Health Med. 2007 Se Oct; 13 (5):66-76.

THE MISSING PHYSIOLOGICAL SYSTEM

The Endocannabinoid System Modulating Levels of Consciousness, Emotions and Likely Dream Contents. Murillo-Rodriguez E1, Pastrana-Trejo JC2, Salas-Crisóstomo M3, de-la-Cruz M, CNS Neurol Disord Drug Targets 2017;16 (4):370-379

David B. Allen, M.D. D. *Survey Shows Low Acceptance of the Science of the ECS* (Endocannabinoid System). Outword Magazine. http://www.outwordmagazine.com/inside-outword/glbt-news/1266-survey-shows-low-acceptance-of-the-science-of-the-ecs-endo cannabinoid-system. Gregory Gerdeman. Biology | Eckerd College. https://www.eckerd.edu/biology/faculty/gerdeman/

THE MEDICAL TRAVESTY

The Endocannabinoid System Modulating Levels of Consciousness, Emoions and Likely Dream Contents., Murillo-Rodriguez E, Pastrana-Tre jo JC,Salas-Crisóstomo M, de-la-Cruz M., CNS Neurol Disord Drug Targets. 2017;16(4):370-379.

Endocannabinoid Signaling and Memory Dynamics: A Synaptic Perspective., Drumond A, Madeira N, Fonseca R., Neurobiol Learn Mem. 2017Feb; 138:62-77

Endocannabinoid Signaling and the Hypothalamic-Pituitary-Adrenal Axis., Hillard CJ, Beatka M, Sarvaideo J., Compr Physiol. 2016 Dec 6;7(1):1-15

*Endocannabinoid System: the Direct and Indirect Involvement in the Memory and Learning Processes-*a Short Review., Kruk-Slomka M, Dzik A,Budzynska B., Mol Neurobiol. 2016 Dec 6.

THE BRAINS BEHIND THE DISCOVERY OF ECS

Endocannabinoid Signaling at the Periphery: 50 Years After THC., Maccarrone M, Bab I, Biro T, Cabral GA, Dey SK, Di Marzo V, Konje JC, Kunos G, Mechoulam R, Pacher P, Sharkey KA, Zimmer A., Trends Pharmacol Sci. 2015 May;36(5):277-96.

The Endocannabinoid System and the Brain., Mechoulam R, Parker LA., Annu Rev Psychol. 2013;64:21-47.

Early Phytocannabinoid Chemistry to Endocannabinoids and Beyond., Mechoulam R, Hanus LO, Pertwee R, Howlett AC.,

ENDOCANNABINOIDS AND THEIR RECEPTORS

Duncan M, Davison JS, Sharkey KA. Review article: *Endocannabinoids and Their Receptors in the Enteric Nervous System.* Aliment Pharmacol Ther. 2005 Oct 15; 22(8):667-83.

Dobovišek L, Hojnik M, Ferk P. *Overlapping molecular pathways between cannabinoid receptors type 1 and 2 and estrogens/androgens on the periphery and their involvement in the pathogenesis of common diseases* (Review). Int J Mol Med. 2016 Dec;38(6):1642-1651.

Svízenská I, Dubový P, Sulcová A. *Cannabinoid receptors 1 and 2 (CB1 and CB2), their distribution, ligands and functional involvement in nervous system structures—a short review.* Pharmacol Biochem Behav. 2008 Oct;90(4):501-11.

Pertwee RG. *The pharmacology of cannabinoid receptors and their ligands: an overview.* Int J Obes (Lond). 2006 Apr;30 Suppl 1:S13-8.

Singh J, Budhiraja S. *Therapeutic potential of cannabinoid receptor ligands: current status.* Methods Find Exp Clin Pharmacol. 2006 Apr;28(3):177-83.

TARGETING MORE THAN JUST CB1 & CB2

Yuan S, Burrell BD. *Endocannabinoid-dependent LTD in a nociceptive synapse requires activation of a presynaptic TRPV-like receptor.* J Neurophysiol. 2010 Nov;104(5):2766-77.

De Petrocellis L, Orlando P, Moriello AS, Aviello G, Stott C, Izzo AA, Di Marzo V. *Cannabinoid actions at TRPV channels: effects on TRPV3 and TRPV4 and their potential relevance to gastrointestinal inflammation.* Acta Physiol (Oxf).2012 Feb;204(2):255-66.
Benze G, Geyer A, Alt-Epping B, Nauck F. [*Treatment of nausea and vomiting with 5HT3 receptor antagonists, steroids, antihistamines, anticholinergics, somatostatinantagonists, benzodiazepines and cannabinoids in palliative care patients : a systematic review*]. Schmerz. 2012 Sep;26(5):481-99.

Sun Y, Alexander SP, Garle MJ, Gibson CL, Hewitt K, Murphy SP, Kendall DA, Bennett AJ. *Cannabinoid activation of PPAR alpha; a novel neuroprotective mechanism.* Br J Pharmacol. 2007 Nov;152(5):734-43.

Russo R, LoVerme J, La Rana G, D'Agostino G, Sasso O, Calignano A, Piomelli D. *Synergistic antinociception by the cannabinoid receptor agonist anandamide and the PPAR-alpha receptor agonist GW7647.* Eur J Pharmacol. 2007 Jul 2;566(1-3):117-9.

Xiong W, Cui T, Cheng K, Yang F, Chen SR, Willenbring D, Guan Y, Pan HL, Ren K, Xu Y, Zhang L. *Cannabinoids suppress inflammatory and neuropathic pain by targeting α3 glycine receptors.* J Exp Med. 2012 Jun 4;209(6):1121-34.

Xiong W, Cheng K, Cui T, Godlewski G, Rice KC, Xu Y, Zhang L. *Cannabinoid potentiation of glycine receptors contributes to cannabis-induced analgesia.* Nat Chem Biol. 2011 May;7(5):296-303.

ANANDAMIDE: MORE THAN JUST BLISS

Fowler CJ. *The cannabinoid system and its pharmacological manipulation--a review, with emphasis upon the uptake and hydrolysis of anandamide.* Fundam Clin Pharmacol. 2006 Dec;20(6):549-62.

Glaser ST, Kaczocha M, Deutsch DG. *Anandamide transport: a critical review.* Life Sci. 2005 Aug 19;77(14):1584-604.

Maccarrone M. *Metabolism of the Endocannabinoid Anandamide: Open Questions after 25 Years.* Front Mol Neurosci. 2017 May 29;10:166.

2-AG: THE WORK HORSE

Kohnz RA, Nomura DK. *Chemical approaches to therapeutically target the metabolism and signaling of the endocannabinoid 2-AG and eicosanoids.* Chem Soc Rev. 2014 Oct 7;43(19):6859-69.

Bari M, Battista N, Fezza F, Gasperi V, Maccarrone M. *New insights into endocannabinoid degradation and its therapeutic potential.* Mini Rev Med Chem. 2006 Mar;6(3):257-68.

Chicca A, Marazzi J, Gertsch J. *The antinociceptive triterpene β-amyrin inhibits 2-arachidonoylglycerol (2-AG) hydrolysis without directly targeting cannabinoid receptors.* Br J Pharmacol. 2012 Dec;167(8):1596-608.

THE SEAT OF CONSCIOUSNESS THE ROLE OF ECS

Endocannabinoid concentrations in hair are associated with PTSD symptom severity, Wilker S, Psychoneuroendocrinology. 2016 May; 67:198-206.

Reductions in circulating endocannabinoid levels in individuals with post-traumatic stress disorder following exposure to the World Trade Center attacks, Hill MN, Psychoneuroendocrinology. 2013 Dec;38(12):2952-61.

Endocannabinoid signaling in hypothalamic circuits regulates arousal from general anesthesia in mice, Haixing Zhong, et al., J ClinInvest.

THE GUT, BRAIN, IMMUNE & ENDOCANNABINOID SYSTEM

Sharkey KA, Wiley JW. *The Role of the Endocannabinoid System in the Brain-Gut Axis.* Gastroenterology. 2016 Aug;151(2):252-66.

Nandini Acharya, *Endocannabinoid system acts as a regulator of immune homeostasis in the gut.*, Proc Natl Acad Sci U S A. 2017 May 9;114(19): 5005–5010

Storr MA, Sharkey KA. The endocannabinoid system and gut-brain signalling. Curr Opin Pharmacol. 2007 Dec;7(6):575-82.

Cluny NL, Reimer RA, Sharkey KA. *Cannabinoid signalling regulates inflammation and energy balance: the importance of the brain-gut axis.* Brain Behav Immun. 2012 Jul;26(5):691-8.

Acharya N, Penukonda S, Shcheglova T, Hagymasi AT, Basu S, Srivastava PK. *Endocannabinoid system acts as a regulator of immune ho-*

meostasis in the gut. Proc Natl Acad Sci U S A. 2017 May 9;114(19):5005-5010.

DiPatrizio NV. *Endocannabinoids in the Gut. Cannabis Cannabinoid* Res. 2016 Feb;1(1):67-77. Epub 2016 Feb 24.

Luft FC. *Endocannabinoids, Just a Gut fFeling.* J Mol Med (Berl). 2007 May;85(5):423-5. Epub 2007 Apr 20.

Pinto L, Capasso R, Di Carlo G, Izzo AA. *Endocannabinoids and the Gut. Prostaglandins Leukot Essent Fatty Acids.* 2002 Feb-Mar;66(2-3):333-41.
Di Marzo V, Piscitelli F. *Gut Feelings About the Endocannabinoid System.,* Neurogastroenterol Motil. 2011 May;23(5):391-8.

Nicholas V. DiPatrizio *Endocannabinoids in the Gut., Cannabis Cannabinoid* Res. 2016; 1(1): 67–77.

Yoo BB., Mazmanian SK. The Enteric Network: *Interactions Between the Immune and Nervous Systems of the Gut.,* Immunity. 2017 Jun20;46(6):910-926.

Powell N., Walker MM., Talley NJ. *The Mucosal Immune System: master regulator of bidirectional gut-brain communications.,.* Nat Rev Gastroenterol Hepatol. 2017 Mar;14(3):143-159.

Dinan TG., Cryan JF. *The Microbiome-Gut-Brain Axis in Health and Disease.,* Gastroenterol Clin North Am. 2017 Mar;46(1):77-89.

ENDOCANNABINOID SYSYTEM & EXERCISE
Stone NL, Millar SA, Herrod PJJ, Barrett DA, Ortori CA, Mellon VA, O'Sullivan SE. *An Analysis of Endocannabinoid Concentrations and Mood Following Singing and Exercise in Healthy Volunteers.* Front Behav Neurosci. 2018 Nov 26;12:269.

Crombie KM, Brellenthin AG, Hillard CJ, Koltyn KF. *Endocannabinoid and Opioid System Interactions in Exercise-Induced Hypoalgesia.* Pain Med. 2018 Jan 1;19(1):118-123.

Brellenthin AG, Crombie KM, Hillard CJ, Koltyn KF. *Endocannabinoid and MoodResponses to Exercise in Adults with Varying Activity Levels.* Med Sci Sports Exerc. 2017 Aug;49(8):1688-1696.

Gamelin FX, Aucouturier J, Iannotti FA, Piscitelli F, Mazzarella E, Aveta T, Leriche M, Dupont E, Cieniewski-Bernard C, Leclair E, Bastide B, Di Marzo V, Heyman E. *Exercise training and high-fat diet elicit endocannabinoid system modifications in the rat hypothalamus and hippocampus.* J Physiol Biochem. 2016 Aug;73(3):335-347.

Gamelin FX, Aucouturier J, Iannotti FA, Piscitelli F, Mazzarella E, Aveta T, Leriche M, Dupont E, Cieniewski-Bernard C, Montel V, Bastide B, Di Marzo V, Heyman E. *Effects of chronic exercise on the endocannabinoid system in Wistar rats with high-fat diet-induced obesity.* J Physiol Biochem. 2016 Jun;72(2):183-99.

Galdino G, Romero T, Silva JF, Aguiar D, Paula AM, Cruz J, Parrella C, Piscitelli F, Duarte I, Di Marzo V, Perez A. *Acute resistance exercise induces antinociception by activation of the endocannabinoid system in rats.* Anesth Analg. 2014 Sep;119(3):702-15.

Galdino G, Romero TR, Silva JF, Aguiar DC, de Paula AM, Cruz JS, Parrella C, Piscitelli F, Duarte ID, Di Marzo V, Perez AC. *The endocannabinoid system mediates aerobic exercise-induced antinociception in rats.* Neuropharmacology. 2014 Feb;77:313-24.

Ferreira-Vieira TH, Bastos CP, Pereira GS, Moreira FA, Massensini AR. *A role for the endocannabinoid system in exercise-induced spatial memory enhancement in mice.* Hippocampus. 2014 Jan;24(1):79-88.

Raichlen DA, Foster AD, Seillier A, Giuffrida A, Gerdeman GL. *Exercise-induced endocannabinoid signaling is modulated by intensity.* Eur J Appl Physiol. 2013 Apr;113(4):869-75.

Heyman E, Gamelin FX, Aucouturier J, Di Marzo V. *The role of the endocannabinoid system in skeletal muscle and metabolic adaptations to exercise: potential implications for the treatment of obesity.* Obes Rev. 2012 Dec;13(12):1110-24.

Raichlen DA, Foster AD, Gerdeman GL, Seillier A, Giuffrida A. *Wired to run: Exercise-induced Endocannabinoid Signaling in Humans and Cursorial Mammals with Implications for the "Runner's High".* J Exp Biol. 2012 Apr 15;215(Pt 8):1331-6.

Feuerecker M, Hauer D, Toth R, Demetz F, Hölzl J, Thiel M, Kaufmann I, Schelling G, Choukèr A. *Effects of exercise stress on the endo-cannabinoid system in humans under field conditions.* Eur J Appl Physiol. 2012 Jul;112(7):2777-81.

Heyman E, Gamelin FX, Goekint M, Piscitelli F, Roelands B, Leclair E, Di Marzo V, Meeusen R. *Intense exercise increases circulating en-*

docannabinoid and BDNF levels in humans--possible implications for reward and depression. Psychoneuroendocrinology. 2012 Jun;37(6):844-51.

Sparling PB, Giuffrida A, Piomelli D, Rosskopf L, Dietrich A. *Exercise activates the endocannabinoid system*. Neuroreport. 2003 Dec 2;14(17):2209-11.

Watkins BA. *Endocannabinoids, Exercise, Pain, and a Path to Health With Aging*. Mol Aspects Med. 2018 Dec;64:68-78.
King-Himmelreich TS, Möser CV, Wolters MC, Schmetzer J, Schreiber Y, Ferreirós N, Russe OQ, Geisslinger G, Niederberger E. *AMPK contributes to aerobic exercise-induced antinociception downstream of endocannabinoids*. Neuropharmacology. 2017 Sep 15;124:134-142.

Thompson Z, Argueta D, Garland T Jr, DiPatrizio N. *Circulating levels of endocannabinoids respond acutely to voluntary exercise, are altered in mice selectively bred for high voluntary wheel running, and differ between the sexes*. Physiol Behav. 2017 Mar 1;170:141-150.

Dietrich A, McDaniel WF. *Endocannabinoids and Exercise*. Br J Sports Med. 2004 Oct;38(5):536-41.

Exercise-induced endocannabinoid signaling is modulated by intensity., Raichlen DA, Foster AD, Seillier A, Giuffrida A, Gerdeman GL., Eur J Appl Physiol. 2013 Apr;113(4):869-75

ENDOCANNABINOID DEFICIENCY

Schlabritz-Loutsevitch N, German N, Ventolini G, Larumbe E, Samson J. *Fetal Syndrome of Endocannabinoid Deficiency (FSECD) In Maternal Obesity*. Med Hypotheses. 2016 Nov;96:35-38.

Russo EB. *Clinical Endocannabinoid Deficiency Reconsidered: Current Research Supports the Theory in Migraine, Fibromyalgia, Irritable Bowel, and Other Treatment-Resistant Syndromes. Cannabis Cannabinoid.* Res. 2016 Jul 1;1(1):154-165.

Patel S, Shonesy BC, Bluett RJ, Winder DG, Colbran RJ. *The Anxiolytic Actions of 2-Arachidonoylglycerol: Converging Evidence From Two Recent Genetic Endocannabinoid Deficiency Models*. Biol Psychiatry. 2016 May 15;79(10):e78-e79.

Bluett RJ, Gamble-George JC, Hermanson DJ, Hartley ND, Marnett LJ, Patel S. *Central anandamide deficiency predicts stress-induced anxiety: behavioral reversal through endocannabinoid augmentation*. Transl Psychiatry. 2014 Jul 8;4:e408.

Smith SC, Wagner MS. *Clinical Endocannabinoid Deficiency (CECD) Revisited: Can this concept explain the therapeutic benefits of cannabis in migraine, fibromyalgia, irritable bowel syndrome and other treatment-resistant conditions?* Neuro Endocrinol Lett. 2014;35(3):198-201.

Schechter M, Weller A, Pittel Z, Gross M, Zimmer A, Pinhasov A. *Endocannabinoid receptor deficiency affects maternal care and alters the dam's hippocampal oxytocin receptor and brain-derived neurotrophic factor expression*. J Neuroendocrinol. 2013 Oct;25(10):898-909.

Russo EB. *Clinical Endocannabinoid Deficiency (CECD): Can this concept explain therapeutic benefits of cannabis in migraine, fibromyalgia, irritable bowel syndrome and other treatment-resistant conditions?* Neuro Endocrinol Lett. 2008 Apr;29(2):192-200.

Russo EB. *Clinical Endocannabinoid Deficiency (CECD): Can this concept explain therapeutic benefits of cannabis in migraine, fibromyalgia, irritable bowel syndrome and other treatment-resistant conditions?* Neuro Endocrinol Lett. 2004 Feb-Apr;25(1-2):31-9.

Hill MN, Lee FS. *Endocannabinoids and Stress Resilience: Is Deficiency Sufficient to Promote Vulnerability?* Biol Psychiatry. 2016 May 15;79(10):792-793.

OMEGA 3 & YOUR ENDOCANNABINIOID SYSTEM

Roy J, Watson JE, Hong IS, Fan TM, Das A. *Antitumorigenic Properties of Omega-3 Endocannabinoid Epoxides*. J Med Chem. 2018 Jul 12;61(13):5569-5579.

McDougle DR, Watson JE, Abdeen AA, Adili R, Caputo MP, Krapf JE, Johnson RW, Kilian KA, Holinstat M, Das A. *Anti-inflammatory ω-3 endocannabinoid epoxides*. Proc Natl Acad Sci U S A. 2017 Jul 25;114(30):E6034-E6043.

Lafourcade M, Larrieu T, Mato S, Duffaud A, Sepers M, Matias I, De Smedt-Peyrusse V, Labrousse VF, Bretillon L, Matute C, Rodríguez-Puertas R, Layé S, Manzoni OJ. *Nutritional omega-3 deficiency abolishes endocannabinoid-mediated neuronal functions*. Nat Neurosci. 2011 Mar;14(3):345-50.

Brown I, Cascio MG, Rotondo D, Pertwee RG, Heys SD, Wahle KW. *Cannabinoids and omega-3/6 endocannabinoids as cell death and anti-cancer modulators*. Prog Lipid Res. 2013 Jan;52(1):80-109.

Brown I, Cascio MG, Wahle KW, Smoum R, Mechoulam R, Ross RA, Pertwee RG, Heys SD. *Cannabinoid receptor-dependent and -independent anti-proliferative effects of omega-3 ethanolamides in androgen receptor-positive and -negative prostate cancer cell lines.* Carcinogenesis. 2010 Sep;31(9):1584-91.

Alharthi N, Christensen P, Hourani W, Ortori C, Barrett DA, Bennett AJ, Chapman V, Alexander SPH. *n-3 polyunsaturated N-acylethanolamines are CB(2) cannabinoid receptor-preferring endocannabinoids.* Biochim Biophys Acta Mol Cell Biol Lipids. 2018 Nov;1863(11):1433-1440.

Larrieu T, Madore C, Joffre C, Layé S. *Nutritional n-3 polyunsaturated fatty acids deficiency alters cannabinoid receptor signaling pathway in the brain and associated anxiety-like behavior in mice.* J Physiol Biochem. 2012 Dec;68(4):671-81.

Rossmeisl M, Pavlisova J, Janovska P, Kuda O, Bardova K, Hansikova J, Svobodova M, Oseeva M, Veleba J, Kopecky J Jr, Zacek P, Fiserova E, Pelikanova T, Kopecky J. *Differential modulation of white adipose tissue endocannabinoid levels by n-3 fatty acids in obese mice and type 2 diabetic patients.* Biochim Biophys Acta Mol Cell Biol Lipids. 2018 Jul;1863(7):712-725.

Dyall SC. *Interplay Between n-3 and n-6 Long-Chain Polyunsaturated Fatty Acids and the Endocannabinoid System in Brain Protection and Repair.* Lipids. 2017 Nov;52(11):885-900.

Thomazeau A, Bosch-Bouju C, Manzoni O, Layé S. *Nutritional n-3 PUFA Deficiency Abolishes Endocannabinoid Gating of Hippocampal Long-Term Potentiation.* Cereb Cortex. 2017 Apr 1;27(4):2571-2579.

Wainwright CL, Michel L. *Endocannabinoid system as a potential mechanism for n-3 long-chain polyunsaturated fatty acid mediated cardiovascular protection.* Proc Nutr Soc. 2013 Nov;72(4):460-9.

Balvers MG, Verhoeckx KC, Bijlsma S, Rubingh CM, Meijerink J, Wortelboer HM, Witkamp RF. *Fish oil and inflammatory status alter the n-3 to n-6 balance of the endocannabinoid and oxylipin metabolomes in mouse plasma and tissues.* Metabolomics. 2012 Dec;8(6):1130-1147.

Oda E. *n-3 Fatty acids and the endocannabinoid system.* Am J Clin Nutr. 2007 Mar;85(3):919; author reply 919-20.

THE ECS IN PAIN & INFLAMMATION

Guerrero-Alba R, Barragán-Iglesias P, González-Hernández A, Valdez-Moráles EE,Granados-Soto V, Condés-Lara M, Rodríguez MG, Marichal-Cancino BA. *Some Prospective Alternatives for Treating Pain: The Endocannabinoid System and Its Putative Receptors GPR18 and GPR55.* Front Pharmacol. 2019 Jan 8;9:1496.

Elliott MB, Ward SJ, Abood ME, Tuma RF, Jallo JI. *Understanding theendocannabinoid system as a modulator of the trigeminal pain response to concussion.* Concussion. 2017 Oct 4;2(4):CNC49.

Masocha W. *Targeting the Endocannabinoid System for Prevention or Treatment of Chemotherapy-Induced Neuropathic Pain: Studies in Animal Models.* Pain Res Manag. 2018 Jul 25;2018:5234943.

Wang Glial J. *Endocannabinoid System in Pain Modulation.* Int J Neurosci. 2018 Aug 7:1-12.

Greco R, Demartini C, Zanaboni AM, Piomelli D, Tassorelli C. *Endocannabinoid System and Migraine Pain: An Update.* Front Neurosci. 2018 Mar 19;12:172.

Barrie N, Manolios N. *The endocannabinoid system in pain and inflammation: Its relevance to rheumatic disease.* Eur J Rheumatol. 2017 Sep;4(3):210-218.

O'Hearn S, Diaz P, Wan BA, DeAngelis C, Lao N, Malek L, Chow E, Blake A. *Modulating the endocannabinoid pathway as treatment for peripheral neuropathic pain: a selected review of preclinical studies.* Ann Palliat Med. 2017 Dec;6(Suppl2):S209-S214.

Ramesh D, D'Agata A, Starkweather AR, Young EE. *Contribution of Endocannabinoid Gene Expression and Genotype on Low Back Pain Susceptibility and Chronicity.* Clin J Pain. 2018 Jan;34(1):8-14.

Sun L, Tai L, Qiu Q, Mitchell R, Fleetwood-Walker S, Joosten EA, Cheung CW. *Endocannabinoid activation of CB(1) receptors contributes to long-lasting reversal of neuropathic pain by repetitive spinal cord stimulation.* Eur J Pain. 2017 May;21(5):804-814

Toguri JT, Caldwell M, Kelly ME. *Turning Down the Thermostat: Modulating the Endocannabinoid System in Ocular Inflammation and Pain.* Front Pharmacol. 2016 Sep 15;7:304.

Malek N, Starowicz K. *Dual-Acting Compounds Targeting Endocannabinoid and Endovanilloid Systems-A Novel Treatment Option for*

Chronic Pain Management. Front Pharmacol. 2016 Aug 17;7:257.

Cajanus K, Holmström EJ, Wessman M, Anttila V, Kaunisto MA, Kalso E. *Effect of endocannabinoid degradation on pain: role of FAAH polymorphisms in experimental and postoperative pain in women treated for breast cancer.* Pain. 2016 Feb;157(2):361-9.

Maldonado R, Baños JE, Cabañero D. *The Endocannabinoid System and Neuropathic Pain.* Pain. 2016 Feb;157 Suppl 1:S23-32.

Corcoran L, Roche M, Finn DP. *The Role of the Brain's Endocannabinoid System in Pain and Its Modulation by Stress.* Int Rev Neurobiol. 2015;125:203-55.

Kaczocha M, Glaser ST, Maher T, Clavin B, Hamilton J, O'Rourke J, Rebecchi M, Puopolo M, Owada Y, Thanos PK. *Fatty acid binding protein deletion suppresses inflammatory pain through endocannabinoid/N-acylethanolamine-dependent mechanisms.* Mol Pain. 2015 Aug 28;11:52.

Cristino L, Luongo L, Imperatore R, Boccella S, Becker T, Morello G, Piscitelli F, Busetto G, Maione S, Di Marzo V. *Orexin-A and Endocannabinoid Activation of the Descending Antinociceptive Pathway Underlies Altered Pain Perception in Leptin Signaling Deficiency.* Neuropsychopharmacology. 2016 Jan;41(2):508-20.

La Porta C, Bura SA, Llorente-Onaindia J, Pastor A, Navarrete F, García-Gutiérrez MS, De la Torre R, Manzanares J, Monfort J, Maldonado R. *Role of the endocannabinoid system in the emotional manifestations of osteoarthritis pain.* Pain. 2015 Oct;156(10):2001-12.

Woodhams SG, Sagar DR, Burston JJ, Chapman V. *The Role of the Endocannabinoid System in Pain.* Handb Exp Pharmacol. 2015;227:119-43.

Ulugöl A. *The endocannabinoid system as a potential therapeutic target for pain modulation.* Balkan Med J. 2014 Jun;31(2):115-20.

La Porta C, Bura SA, Negrete R, Maldonado R. *Involvement of the endocannabinoid system in osteoarthritis pain.* Eur J Neurosci. 2014 Feb;39(3):485-500.

No more pain upon Gq-protein-coupled receptor activation: Role of endocannabinoids. Eur J Neurosci. 2016 Apr;43(7):991.

Azim S, Nicholson J, Rebecchi MJ, Galbavy W, Feng T, Reinsel R, Volkow ND, Benveniste H, Kaczocha M. *Endocannabinoids and acute pain after total knee arthroplasty.* Pain. 2015 Feb;156(2):341-347.

Hu SS, Ho YC, Chiou LC. *No more pain upon Gq-protein-coupled receptor activation: role of endocannabinoids.* Eur J Neurosci. 2014 Feb;39(3):467-84.

Luongo L, Maione S, Di Marzo V. *Endocannabinoids and neuropathic pain: focuson neuron-glia and endocannabinoid-neurotrophin interactions.* Eur J Neurosci. 2014 Feb;39(3):401-8.

Zogopoulos P, Vasileiou I, Patsouris E, Theocharis SE. *The role of endocannabinoids in pain modulation.* Fundam Clin Pharmacol. 2013 Feb;27(1):64-80.

Lovinger DM. *Endocannabinoids rein in pain outside the brain.* Nat Neurosci. 2010 Oct;13(10):1155-6.

Pesce M, Esposito G, Sarnelli G. *Endocannabinoids in the treatment of gasytrointestinal inflammation and symptoms.* Curr Opin Pharmacol. 2018 Dec;43:81-86.

Dickson I. *Endocannabinoids counterbalance intestinal inflammation.* Nat Rev Gastroenterol Hepatol. 2018 Nov;15(11):656-657.

Krustev E, Muley MM, McDougall JJ. *Endocannabinoids inhibit neurogenic inflammation in murine joints by a non-canonical cannabinoid receptor mechanism.* Neuropeptides. 2017 Aug;64:131-135.

Turcotte C, Chouinard F, Lefebvre JS, Flamand N. *Regulation of inflammation by cannabinoids, the endocannabinoids 2-arachidonoyl-glycerol and arachidonoyl-ethanolamide, and their metabolites.* J Leukoc Biol. 2015 Jun;97(6):1049-70.

Krishnan G, Chatterjee N. *Endocannabinoids alleviate proinflammatory conditions by modulating innate immune response in muller glia during inflammation.* Glia. 2012 Nov;60(11):1629-45.

Endocannabinoid Research Group, De Filippis D, D'Amico A, Cipriano M, Petrosino S, Orlando P, Di Marzo V, Iuvone T. *Levels of endocannabinoids and palmitoylethanolamide and their pharmacological manipulation in chronic granulomatous inflammation in rats.* Pharmacol Res. 2010 Apr;61(4):321-8.

Burstein SH, Zurier RB. *Cannabinoids, endocannabinoids, and related analogs in inflammation.* AAPS J. 2009 Mar;11(1):109-19.

Marchalant Y, Brothers HM, Wenk GL. *Inflammation and aging: can endocannabinoids help?* Biomed Pharmacother. 2008 Apr-May;62(4):212-7. Grill M, Hasenoehrl C, Kienzl M, Kargl J, Schicho R. *Cellular localization and regulation of receptors and enzymes of the endocannabinoid system in intestinal and systemic inflammation.* Histochem Cell Biol. 2019 Jan;151(1):5-20.

Barrie N, Manolios N. *The endocannabinoid system in pain and inflammation: Its relevance to rheumatic disease.* Eur J Rheumatol. 2017 Sep;4(3):210-218.

Crowe MS, Nass SR, Gabella KM, Kinsey SG. *The endocannabinoid system modulates stress, emotionality, and inflammation.* Brain Behav Immun. 2014 Nov;42:1-5.

De Laurentiis A, Araujo HA, Rettori V. *Role of the endocannabinoid system in the neuroendocrine responses to inflammation.* Curr Pharm Des. 2014;20(29):4697-706.

Witkamp R, Meijerink J. *The endocannabinoid system: an emerging key player in inflammation.* Curr Opin Clin Nutr Metab Care. 2014 Mar;17(2):130-8.

THE ECS & SLEEP

Murillo-Rodríguez E, Machado S, Rocha NB, Budde H, Yuan TF, Arias-Carrión O. *Revealing the role of the endocannabinoid system modulators, SR141716A, URB597 and VDM-11, in sleep homeostasis.* Neuroscience. 2016 Dec 17;339:433-449.

Pava MJ, Makriyannis A, Lovinger DM. *Endocannabinoid Signaling Regulates Sleep Stability.* PLoS One. 2016 Mar 31;11(3):e0152473.

Pava MJ, Hartford CR, Blanco-Centurion C, Shiromani PJ, Woodward JJ. *Endocannabinoid Modulation of Cortical up-states and NREM Sleep.* PLoS One. 2014 Feb 10;9(2):e88672.

Méndez-Díaz M, Caynas-Rojas S, Arteaga Santacruz V, Ruiz-Contreras AE, Aguilar-Roblero R, Prospéro-García O. *Entopeduncular nucleus endocannabinoid system modulates sleep-waking cycle and mood in rats.* Pharmacol Biochem Behav.2013 Jun;107:29-35.

Murillo-Rodríguez E, Palomero-Rivero M, Millán-Aldaco D, Di Marzo V. *The administration of endocannabinoid uptake inhibitors OMDM-2 or VDM-11 promote sleep and decreases extracellular levels of dopamine in rats.* Physiol Behav. 2013 Jan 17;109:88-95.

Murillo-Rodriguez E, Poot-Ake A, Arias-Carrion O, Pacheco-Pantoja E, Fuente-Ortegon Ade L, Arankowsky-Sandoval G. *The emerging role of the endocannabinoid system in the sleep-wake cycle modulation.* Cent Nerv Syst Agents Med Chem. 2011 Sep 1;11(3):189-96.

Wang LY, Yang T, Qian W, Hou XH. [*Effects of central endocannabinoid system on visceral hyposensitivity induced by rapid eye movement sleep deprivation: Experiment with rats*]. Zhonghua Yi Xue Za Zhi. 2009 Mar 3;89(8):559-63. Chinese.

Prospéro-García O, Amancio-Belmont O, Becerril Meléndez AL, Ruiz-Contreras AE, Méndez-Díaz M. *Endocannabinoids and Sleep.* Neurosci Biobehav Rev. 2016 Dec;71:671-679.

Cedernaes J, Fanelli F, Fazzini A, Pagotto U, Broman JE, Vogel H, Dickson SL, Schiöth HB, Benedict C. *Sleep restriction alters plasma endocannabinoids concentrations before but not after exercise in humans.* Psychoneuroendocrinology. 2016 Dec;74:258-268.

Scheer FA. *Hungry for Sleep: A Role for Endocannabinoids?* Sleep. 2016 Mar 1;39(3):495-6.

Murillo-Rodríguez E. [*The modulatory role of endocannabinoids in sleep*]. Rev Neurol. 2008 Feb 1-15;46(3):160-6.

ECS & BONE HEALTH

Beguier F, Epelman S. *Endocannabinoid signalling: Bone marrow monocytes and neutrophils follow their nose into ischemic tissue.* Cardiovasc Res. 2019 Jan 10.

Pura M, Va uga P. [*The endocannabinoid system and bone*]. Vnitr Lek. Fall 2016;62(9 Suppl 3):99-102. Czech. PubMed PMID: 27734700.

Zimmer A. *A collaboration investigating endocannabinoid signalling in brain and bone.* J Basic Clin Physiol Pharmacol. 2016 May 1;27(3):229-35.

Rossi F, Siniscalco D, Luongo L, De Petrocellis L, Bellini G, Petrosino S,Torella M, Santoro C, Nobili B, Perrotta S, Di Marzo V, Maione S. *The endovanilloid/endocannabinoid system in human osteoclasts: possible involvement in bone formation and resorption.* Bone. 2009 Mar;44(3):476-84.
Rossi F, Bellini G, Luongo L, Torella M, Mancusi S, De Petrocellis L, Petrosino S, Siniscalco D, Orlando P, Scafuro M, Colacurci N, Perrotta S, Nobili, B, Di Marzo V, Maione S; *Endocannabinoid Research Group (ERG), Italy. The Endovanilloid/Endocannabinoid System: A New Potential Target for Osteoporosis Therapy.* Bone. 2011 May 1;48(5):997-1007.

Smith M, Wilson R, O'Brien S, Tufarelli C, Anderson SI, O'Sullivan SE. *The Effects of the Endocannabinoids Anandamide and 2-Arachidonoylglycerol on Human Osteoblast Proliferation and Differentiation.* PLoS One. 2015 Sep 28;10(9):e0136546.

Whyte LS, Ford L, Ridge SA, Cameron GA, Rogers MJ, Ross RA. *Cannabinoids and bone: endocannabinoids modulate human osteoclast function in vitro.* Br J Pharmacol. 2012 Apr;165(8):2584-97.

Bab I, Ofek O, Tam J, Rehnelt J, Zimmer A. *Endocannabinoids and the regulation of bone metabolism.* J Neuroendocrinol. 2008 May;20 Suppl 1:69-74.

Zhu M, Yu B, Bai J, Wang X, Guo X, Liu Y, Lin J, Hu S, Zhang W, Tao Y, Hu C, Yang H, Xu Y, Geng D. *Cannabinoid receptor 2 agonist prevents local and systemic inflammatory bone destruction in rheumatoid arthritis.* J Bone Miner Res. 2018 Dec 3.

Jiang H, Wu Y, Valverde P, Murray D, Tang J, Yao Q, Han Q, Zhang J, Zhang L, Sui L, Tang Y, Tu Q, Chen J. Central adiponectin induces trabecular bone mass partly through epigenetic downregulation of cannabinoid receptor CB1. J Cell Physiol. 2019 May;234(5):7062-7069.

Deis S, Srivastava RK, Ruiz de Azua I, Bindila L, Baraghithy S, Lutz B, Bab I,Tam J. *Age-related regulation of bone formation by the sympathetic cannabinoid CB1 receptor.* Bone. 2018 Mar;108:34-42.

Wang B, Lian K, Li J, Mei G. *Restoration of osteogenic differentiation by over expression of cannabinoid receptor 2 in bone marrow mesenchymal stem cells isolated from osteoporotic patients.* Exp Ther Med. 2018 Jan;15(1):357-364.

Marino S, Idris AI. *Emerging therapeutic targets in cancer induced bone disease: A focus on the peripheral type 2 cannabinoid receptor.* Pharmacol Res.2017 May;119:391-403.

Sun YX, Xu AH, Yang Y, Zhang JX, Yu AW. Activation of cannabinoid receptor 2 enhances osteogenic differentiation of bone marrow derived mesenchymal stem cells. Biomed Res Int. 2015;2015:874982.

Gowran A, McKayed K, Campbell VA. *The cannabinoid receptor type 1 is essential for mesenchymal stem cell survival and differentiation: implications for bone health.* Stem Cells Int. 2013;2013:796715.

Sophocleous A, Landao-Bassonga E, Van't Hof RJ, Idris AI, Ralston SH. *The type 2 cannabinoid receptor regulates bone mass and ovariectomy-induced bone loss by affecting osteoblast differentiation and bone formation.* Endocrinology. 2011 Jun;152(6):2141-9.

ECS STRESS/ANXIETY

Chen Z, Kenny PJ. *Endocannabinoid Signaling in the Habenula Regulates Adaptive Responses to Stress.* Biol Psychiatry. 2018 Oct 15;84(8):553-554.

Wirz L, Reuter M, Felten A, Schwabe L. *An endocannabinoid receptor polymorphism modulates affective processing under stress.* Soc Cogn Affect Neurosci. 2018 Nov 8;13(11):1177-1189.

Micale V, Drago F. *Endocannabinoid system, stress and HPA axis.* Eur J Pharmacol. 2018 Sep 5;834:230-239.

Ney LJ, Matthews A, Bruno R, Felmingham KL. *Modulation of the endocannabinoid system by sex hormones: Implications for posttraumatic stress disorder.* Neurosci Biobehav Rev. 2018 Nov;94:302-320.

Berger AL, Henricks AM, Lugo JM, Wright HR, Warrick CR, Sticht MA, Morena M, Bonilla I, Laredo SA, Craft RM, Parsons LH, Grandes PR, Hillard CJ, Hill MN, McLaughlin RJ. *The Lateral Habenula Directs Coping Styles Under Conditions of Stress via Recruitment of the Endocannabinoid System.* Biol Psychiatry. 2018 Oct15;84(8):611-623.

Atsak P, Morena M, Schoenmaker C, Tabak E, Oomen CA, Jamil S, Hill MN, Roozendaal B. *Glucocorticoid-endocannabinoid uncoupling mediates fear suppression deficits after early - Life stress.* Psychoneuroendocrinology. 2018 May;91:41-49.

Krug RG 2nd, Lee HB, El Khoury LY, Sigafoos AN, Petersen MO, Clark KJ. *The endocannabinoid gene faah2a modulates stress-associated behavior in zebra fish.* PLoS One. 2018 Jan 5;13(1):e0190897.

Morena M, Berardi A, Colucci P, Palmery M, Trezza V, Hill MN, Campolongo P. *Enhancing Endocannabinoid Neurotransmission Augments The Efficacy of Extinction Training and Ameliorates Traumatic Stress-Induced Behavioral Alterations in Rats.* Neuropsychopharmacology. 2018 May;43(6):1284-1296.

Surkin PN, Gallino SL, Luce V, Correa F, Fernandez-Solari J, De Laurentiis A. *Pharmacological augmentation of endocannabinoid signaling reduces the neuroendocrine response to stress.* Psychoneuroendocrinology. 2018 Jan;87:131-140.

Hill MN, Campolongo P, Yehuda R, Patel S. *Integrating Endocannabinoid Signaling and Cannabinoids into the Biology and Treatment of Posttraumatic Stress Disorder.* Neuropsychopharmacology. 2018 Jan;43(1):80-102.

Bluett RJ, Báldi R, Haymer A, Gaulden AD, Hartley ND, Parrish WP, Baechle J, Marcus DJ, Mardam-Bey R, Shonesy BC, Uddin MJ, Marnett LJ, Mackie K, Colbran RJ, Winder DG, Patel S. *Endocannabinoid signalling modulates susceptibility to traumatic stress exposure.* Nat Commun. 2017 Mar 28;8:14782.

Di S, Itoga CA, Fisher MO, Solomonow J, Roltsch EA, Gilpin NW, Tasker JG., *Acute Stress Suppresses Synaptic Inhibition and Increases Anxiety via Endocannabinoid Release in the Basolateral Amygdala.* J Neurosci. 2016 Aug 10;36(32):8461-70.

Berardi A, Schelling G, Campolongo P. *The endocannabinoid system and Post Traumatic Stress Disorder (PTSD): From preclinical findings to innovative therapeutic approaches in clinical settings.* Pharmacol Res. 2016 Sep;111:668-678.

Bosch-Bouju C, Larrieu T, Linders L, Manzoni OJ, Layé S., *Endocannabinoid-Mediated Plasticity in Nucleus Accumbens Controls Vulnerability to Anxiety after Social Defeat Stress.* Cell Rep. 2016 Aug 2;16(5):1237-1242.

Lee TT, Gorzalka BB. *Evidence for a Role of Adolescent Endocannabinoid Signaling in Regulating HPA Axis Stress Responsivity and Emotional Behavior Development.* Int Rev Neurobiol. 2015;125:49-84.

Lutz B, Marsicano G, Maldonado R, Hillard CJ. *The endocannabinoid system in guarding against fear, anxiety and stress.* Nat Rev Neurosci. 2015 Dec;16(12):705-18.

Lim J, Igarashi M, Jung KM, Butini S, Campiani G, Piomelli D. *Endocannabinoid Modulation of Predator Stress-Induced Long-Term Anxiety in Rats.* Neuropsychopharmacology. 2016 Apr;41(5):1329-39.

Morena M, Patel S, Bains JS, Hill MN. *Neurobiological Interactions Between Stress and the Endocannabinoid System.* Neuropsychopharmacology. 2016 Jan;41(1):80-102.

Yin AQ, Wang F, Zhang X. *Integrating endocannabinoid signaling in the regulation of anxiety and depression.* Acta Pharmacol Sin. 2018 Jul 12.

Bedse G, Bluett RJ, Patrick TA, Romness NK, Gaulden AD, Kingsley PJ, Plath N, Marnett LJ, Patel S. *Therapeutic endocannabinoid augmentation for mood and anxiety disorders: comparative profiling of FAAH, MAGL and dual inhibitors.,* Transl Psychiatry. 2018 Apr 26;8(1):92.

Lisboa SF, Gomes FV, Terzian AL, Aguiar DC, Moreira FA, Resstel LB, Guimarães FS. *The Endocannabinoid System and Anxiety.* Vitam Horm. 2017;103:193-279.

Bedse G, Hartley ND, Neale E, Gaulden AD, Patrick TA, Kingsley PJ, Uddin MJ, Plath N, Marnett LJ, Patel S., *Functional Redundancy Between Canonical Endocannabinoid Signaling Systems in the Modulation of Anxiety.* Biol Psychiatry. 2017 Oct 1;82(7):488-499.

Morena M, Leitl KD, Vecchiarelli HA, Gray JM, Campolongo P, Hill MN. *Emotional arousal state influences the ability of amygdalar endocannabinoid signaling to modulate anxiety.* Neuropharmacology. 2016 Dec;111:59-69.

Di S, Itoga CA, Fisher MO, Solomonow J, Roltsch EA, Gilpin NW, Tasker JG., *Acute Stress Suppresses Synaptic Inhibition and Increases Anxiety via Endocannabinoid Release in the Basolateral Amygdala.* J Neurosci. 2016 Aug10;36(32):8461-70.

Lutz B, Marsicano G, Maldonado R, Hillard CJ. *The Endocannabinoid System in Guarding Against Fear, Anxiety and Stress.* Nat Rev

Neurosci. 2015 Dec;16(12):705-18.

Korem N, Zer-Aviv TM, Ganon-Elazar E, Abush H, Akirav I. *Targeting the endocannabinoid system to treat anxiety-related disorders.* J Basic Clin Physiol Pharmacol. 2016 May 1;27(3):193-202.

Jenniches I, Ternes S, Albayram O, Otte DM, Bach K, Bindila L, Michel K, Lutz B, Bilkei-Gorzo A, Zimmer A., *Anxiety, Stress, and Fear Response in Mice With Reduced Endocannabinoid Levels.* Biol Psychiatry. 2016 May 15;79(10):858-868.

Qin Z, Zhou X, Pandey NR, Vecchiarelli HA, Stewart CA, Zhang X, Lagace DC, Brunel JM, Béïque JC, Stewart AF, Hill MN, Chen HH. *Chronic stress induces anxiety via an amygdalar cascade that impairs endocannabinoid signaling.* Neuron. 2015 Mar 18;85(6):1319-31.

Shonesy BC, Bluett RJ, Ramikie TS, Báldi R, Hermanson DJ, Kingsley PJ, Marnett LJ, Winder DG, Colbran RJ, Patel S. *Genetic disruption of 2-arachidonoylglycerol synthesis reveals a key role for endocannabinoid signaling in anxiety modulation.* Cell Rep. 2014 Dec 11;9(5):1644-1653.

Bluett RJ, Gamble-George JC, Hermanson DJ, Hartley ND, Marnett LJ, Patel S., *Central anandamide deficiency predicts stress-induced anxiety: behavioral reversal through endocannabinoid augmentation.* Transl Psychiatry. 2014 Jul 8;4:e408.

Almeida-Santos AF, Gobira PH, Rosa LC, Guimaraes FS, Moreira FA, Aguiar DC., *Modulation of anxiety-like behavior by the endocannabinoid 2-arachidonoylglycerol(2-AG) in the dorsolateral periaqueductal gray.* Behav Brain Res. 2013 Sep1;252:10-7.

Hakimizadeh E, Oryan S, Hajizadeh Moghaddam A, Shamsizadeh A, Roohbakhsh A. *Endocannabinoid System and TRPV1 Receptors in the Dorsal Hippocampus of the Rats Modulate Anxiety-like Behaviors.* Iran J Basic Med Sci. 2012 May;15(3):795-802.

Fogaça MV, Aguiar DC, Moreira FA, Guimarães FS. *The endocannabinoid and endovanilloid systems interact in the rat prelimbic medial prefrontal cortex to control anxiety-like behavior.* Neuropharmacology. 2012 Aug;63(2):202-10.

Ruehle S, Rey AA, Remmers F, Lutz B. *The endocannabinoid system in anxiety, fear memory and habituation.* J Psychopharmacol. 2012 Jan;26(1):23-39.

Saito VM, Wotjak CT, Moreira FA. [*Pharmacological exploitation of the endocannabinoid system: new perspectives for the treatment of depression and anxiety disorders?*]. Braz J Psychiatry. 2010 May;32 Suppl 1:S7-14.

Hill MN, Gorzalka BB. *The endocannabinoid system and the treatment of mood and anxiety disorders.* CNS Neurol Disord Drug Targets. 2009 Dec;8(6):451-8.

Patel S, Hillard CJ. *Role of endocannabinoid signaling in anxiety and depression.* Curr Top Behav Neurosci. 2009;1:347-71.

Domschke K, Zwanzger P. *GABAergic and endocannabinoid dysfunction in anxiety - future therapeutic targets?* Curr Pharm Des. 2008;14(33):3508-17.

ECS, PHYTOCANNABINOIDS & CANCER

Fraguas-Sánchez AI, Martín-Sabroso C, Torres-Suárez AI. *Insights into the effects of the endocannabinoid system in cancer: a review.* Br J Pharmacol. 2018 Jul;175(13):2566-2580.

Khan MI, Sobocińska AA, Czarnecka AM, Król M, Botta B, Szczylik C. *The Therapeutic Aspects of the Endocannabinoid System (ECS) for Cancer and their Development: From Nature to Laboratory.* Curr Pharm Des. 2016;22(12):1756-66.

Chen L, Chen H, Li Y, Li L, Qiu Y, Ren J. *Endocannabinoid and ceramide levels are altered in patients with colorectal cancer.* Oncol Rep. 2015 Jul;34(1):447-54.

Ayakannu T, Taylor AH, Willets JM, Konje JC. *The evolving role of the endocannabinoid system in gynaecological cancer.* Hum Reprod Update. 2015 Jul-Aug;21(4):517-35.

Maccarrone M. *Endocannabinoid Signaling in Cancer: A Rather Complex Puzzle.* Trends Pharmacol Sci. 2013 Aug;34(8):426-7.

Pisanti S, Picardi P, D'Alessandro A, Laezza C, Bifulco M. *The Endocannabinoid Signaling System in Cancer.* Trends Pharmacol Sci. 2013 May;34(5):273-82.

Díaz-Laviada I. *The Endocannabinoid System in Prostate Cancer.* Nat Rev Urol. 2011 Sep 13;8(10):553-61. doi: 10.1038/nrurol.2011.130.

Grimaldi C, Capasso A. *The Endocannabinoid System in the Cancer Therapy: An Overview.* Curr Med Chem. 2011;18(11):1575-83.

Guindon J, Hohmann AG. *The Endocannabinoid System and Cancer: Therapeutic Implication.* Br J Pharmacol. 2011 Aug;163(7):1447-63.

Fowler CJ, Gustafsson SB, Chung SC, Persson E, Jacobsson SO, Bergh A. *Targeting the endocannabinoid system for the treatment of cancer--a practical view.* Curr Top Med Chem. 2010;10(8):814-27.

Alpini G, Demorrow S. *Changes in the endocannabinoid system may give insight into new and effective treatments for cancer.* Vitam Horm. 2009;81:469-85.

Pisanti S, Bifulco M. *Endocannabinoid system modulation in cancer biology and therapy.* Pharmacol Res. 2009 Aug;60(2):107-16.

U.S. Cancer Statistics Working Group. United States Cancer Statistics: *1999-2014 Incidence and Mortality Web-based Report.* Atlanta: U.S. Department of Health and Human Services, Centers for Disease Control and Prevention and National Cancer Institute;2017. Available at: www.cdc.gov/uscs.

Chakravarti B, Ravi J, Ganju RK (2014). *Cannabinoids as therapeutic agents in cancer: current status and future implications.* Oncotarget. 5(15):5852-72.

Massi P, Vaccani A, Bianchessi S, Costa B, Macchi P, Parolaro D (2006). *The non-psychoactive cannabidiol triggers caspase activation and oxidative stress in human glioma cells.* Cell Mol Life Sci. 63(17):2057-66.

Massi P, Vaccani A, Ceruti S, Colomba, Abbracchio MP, Parolaro D. *Antitumor effects of cannabidiol, a nonpsychoactive cannabinoid, human glioma cell lines.* J Pharmacol. 2004;308(3):838-45.

Massi P, Vaccani A, Bianchessi S, Costa B, Macchi P, Parolaro D (2006). *The non-psychoactive cannabidiol triggers caspase activation and oxidative stress in human glioma cells.* Cell Mol Life Sci. 63(17):2057-66.

Ramer R, Heinemann K, Merkord J, Rohde H, Salamon A, Linnebacher M, Hinz B (2012). *COX-2 and PPAR-γconfer cannabidiol-induced apoptosis of human lung cancer cells.* Mol Cancer Ther. 12(1):69-82.

McKallip RJ, Jia W, Schlomer J, Warren JW, Nagarkatti PS, Nagarkatti M (2006). *Cannabidiol-induced apoptosis in human leukemia cells: A novel role of cannabidiol in the regulation of p22phox and Nox4 expression.* Mol Pharmacol. 70(3):897-908.

Lukhele ST, Motadi LR. *Cannabidiol rather than Cannabis sativa extracts inhibit cell growth and induce apoptosis in cervical cancer cells.* BMC Complement Altern Med. 2016 Sep 1;16(1):335.

Morelli MB, Offidani M, Alesiani F, Discepoli G, Liberati S, Olivieri A, Santoni M, Santoni G, Leoni P, Nabissi M. *The effects of cannabidiol and its synergism with bortezomib in multiple myeloma cell lines. A role for transient receptor potential vanilloid type-2.* Int J Cancer. 2014 Jun 1;134(11):2534-46.

Ramer R, Fischer S, Haustein M, Manda K, Hinz B (2014). *Cannabinoids inhibit angiogenic capacities of endothelial cells via release of tissue inhibitor of matrix metalloproteinases-1 from lung cancer cells.* Biochem Pharmacol.91(2):202-16.

McAllister SD, Christian RT, Horowitz MP, Garcia A, Desprez PY (2007). *Cannabidiol as a novel inhibitor of Id-1 gene expression in aggressive breast cancer cells.* Mol Cancer 6(11):2921-7.

McAllister SD, Murase R, Christian RT, Lau D, Zielinski AJ, Allison J, Almanza C, Pakdel A, Lee J, Limbad C, Liu Y, Debs RJ, MooreDH, Desprez PY (2011). *Pathways mediating the effects of cannabidiol on the reduction of breast cancer cell proliferation, invasion, and metastasis.* 129(1):37- 47.

Arnold JC, Hone P, Holland ML, Allen JD (2012). *CB2 and TRPV1 receptors mediate cannabinoid actions on MDR1 expression in multi drug resistant cells.* Pharmacol Rep. 64(3):751-7.

Holland ML, Lau DT, Allen JD, Arnold JC (2007). *The multidrug transporter ABCG2 (BCRP) is inhibited by plant-derived cannabinoids.* Br J Pharmacol. 152(5):815-24.

Holland ML, Allen JD, Arnold JC (2008). Interaction of plant cannabinoids with the multidrug transporter ABCC1 (MRP1). Eur JPharmacol. 591(1-3):128-31.

Sharkey KA, Darmani NA, Parker LA. *Regulation of nausea and vomiting by cannabinoids and the endocannabinoid system.* EurJ Pharmacol. 722:134-46.

Ward SJ, McAllister SD, Kawamura R, Murase R, Neelakantan H, Walker EA. *Cannabidiol inhibits paclitaxel-induced neuropathic pain through 5-HT(1A) receptors without diminishing nervous system function or chemotherapy efficacy.* Br J Pharmacol. 2014Feb;171(3):636-45.

ECS & EYE HEALTH

Nadolska K, Goś R. [*The role of endocannabinoid system in physiological and pathological processes in the eye*]. Klin Oczna. 2008;110(10-12):392-6.

Toguri JT, Caldwell M, Kelly ME. *Turning Down the Thermostat: Modulating the Endocannabinoid System in Ocular Inflammation and Pain.* Front Pharmacol. 2016 Sep 15;7:304.

Cairns EA, Toguri JT, Porter RF, Szczesniak AM, Kelly ME. *Seeing over the horizon - targeting the endocannabinoid system for the treatment of ocular disease.* J Basic Clin Physiol Pharmacol. 2016 May 1;27(3):253-65.

Cairns EA, Baldridge WH, Kelly ME. *The Endocannabinoid System as a Therapeutic Target in Glaucoma.* Neural Plast. 2016;2016:9364091.

Schwitzer T, Schwan R, Angioi-Duprez K, Giersch A, Laprevote V. *The Endocannabinoid System in the Retina: From Physiology to Practical and Therapeutic Applications.* Neural Plast. 2016;2016:2916732.

Bouchard JF, Casanova C, Cécyre B, Redmond WJ. *Expression and Function of the Endocannabinoid System in the Retina and the Visual Brain.* Neural Plast. 2016;2016:9247057.

Nucci C, Gasperi V, Tartaglione R, Cerulli A, Terrinoni A, Bari M, De Simone C, Agrò AF, Morrone LA, Corasaniti MT, Bagetta G, Maccarrone M. *Involvement of the endocannabinoid system in retinal damage after high intraocular pressure-induced ischemia in rats.* Invest Ophthalmol Vis Sci. 2007 Jul;48(7):2997-3004.

Miller S, Leishman E, Hu SS, Elghouche A, Daily L, Murataeva N, Bradshaw H, Straiker A. *Harnessing the Endocannabinoid 2-Arachidonoylglycerol to Lower Intraocular Pressure in a Murine Model.* Invest Ophthalmol Vis Sci. 2016 Jun 1;57(7):3287-96.

Laine K, Järvinen K, Mechoulam R, Breuer A, Järvinen T. *Comparison of the enzymatic stability and intraocular pressure effects of 2-arachidonylglycerol and noladin ether, a novel putative endocannabinoid.* Invest Ophthalmol Vis Sci. 2002 Oct;43(10):3216-22.

ECS & NEUROLOGICAL HEALTH

Martínez-Pinilla E, Aguinaga D, Navarro G, Rico AJ, Oyarzábal J, Sánchez-Arias JA, Lanciego JL, Franco R. *Targeting CB(1) and GPR55 Endocannabinoid Receptors as a Potential Neuroprotective Approach for Parkinson's Disease.* Mol Neurobiol. 2019 Jan 28.

Mounsey RB, Mustafa S, Robinson L, Ross RA, Riedel G, Pertwee RG, Teismann P. *Increasing levels of the endocannabinoid 2-AG is neuroprotective in the 1-methyl-4-phenyl-1,2,3,6-tetrahydropyridine mouse model of Parkinson's disease.* Exp Neurol. 2015 Nov;273:36-44.

Pisani V, Madeo G, Tassone A, Sciamanna G, Maccarrone M, Stanzione P, Pisani A. *Homeostatic changes of the endocannabinoid system in Parkinson's disease.* Mov Disord. 2011 Feb 1;26(2):216-22.

Di Filippo M, Picconi B, Tozzi A, Ghiglieri V, Rossi A, Calabresi P. *The Endocannabinoid System in Parkinson's Disease.* Curr Pharm Des. 2008;14(23):2337-47.